F

to

Powerful
techniques
to lead you to
kindness

Quarto

First published in 2025 by Leaping Hare Press,
an imprint of The Quarto Group.
One Triptych Place
London, SE1 9SH,
United Kingdom
T (0)20 7700 9000
www.Quarto.com

EEA Representation, WTS Tax d.o.o., Žanova ulica 3, 4000
Kranj, Slovenia
www.wts-tax.si

A catalogue record for this book is available from the British
Library.

ISBN 978-1-83600-857-6
Ebook ISBN 978-1-83600-858-3

10 9 8 7 6 5 4 3 2 1

Text designed and typeset by Dinah Drazin

Editorial Director: Monica Perdoni
Commissioning Editor: Sophie Lazar
Editor: Katerina Menhennet
Senior Designer: Renata Latipova
Senior Production Controller: Rohana Yusof

Printed in the UK CPI092025

MIX
Paper | Supporting
responsible forestry
FSC
www.fsc.org   FSC® C013604

Find Your Path *to* Compassion

Powerful
techniques
to lead you to
kindness

Sally Warren

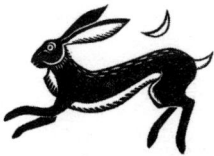

Leaping Hare Press

Dedication

For Marcus and Edward

Contents

Introduction

This book is about compassion and how you can try to develop and practise it to improve your life and the lives of those around you. Compassion is a powerful force for good which can help us to navigate life's complexities and challenges. This book is a self-help manual with simple advice, tips and exercises that you can use at home. It is not an exhaustive study of compassion. We will explore what compassion is, how it affects our minds and bodies, how it evolved, how we develop compassion as children and what barriers can prevent us from being able to practise it. Once we know what these are, we are better placed to overcome them. We will also look at self-compassion: the act of being kinder to ourselves when life gets tough.

'Love and compassion are necessities, not luxuries.
Without them, humanity cannot survive.'

TENZIN GYATSO
The 14th Dalai Lama[1]

Without compassion, the world would be a grim, desolate place. Think about it for a moment. There would be minimal incentive to help our fellow citizens beyond self-interest. The sick and elderly would be left to die, the homeless ignored. The whole fabric of society as we know it would be at risk. Compassion is a value that informs many of the institutions that define our civilization. International institutions in the fields of health, education and justice have compassion at their core. Without compassion, our lives would be brutal, unforgiving, cruel.

Fortunately, there is a lot of compassion around. Think of the people who give their time to volunteer at organizations like the Samaritans, all the people who donate to charity, all the professionals who work for free to help those who are without means to pay. According to the Charities Aid Foundation, 4.3 billion people around the world gave money, time, or helped someone they didn't know in 2023. That is the equivalent to 73 per cent of the world's adult population.

A great example of compassion, or rather someone learning compassion, was formulated by Charles Dickens, the great nineteenth-century English novelist. He created an unforgettable character in Ebenezer Scrooge, the cold-hearted miser in *A Christmas Carol*.[2] Scrooge is preoccupied with money and work; he is selfish, rude, isolated and seemingly completely incapable of kindness or compassion. He doesn't care or concern himself with other people and is certainly not moved by the poverty that surrounds him. Although wealthy, he will only allow his employee Bob Cratchit one piece of coal to warm his office. When asked, he refuses to make a donation to the poor and destitute. Although Scrooge sees people suffering around him, he doesn't care. He has no compassion.

Scrooge is shown the error of his ways in a single night thanks to the visits of the Ghosts of Christmas Past, Christmas Present and Christmas Yet to Come. The following morning, Scrooge is a new person, a compassionate person, who decides to use his wealth to help the poor.

We may not all learn to be compassionate by seeing fantastical ghosts showing us our past, present and future, but *A Christmas Carol* does show us that people can change. And that is what this book is for – to help you reflect on how you might be more compassionate in your life.

As a psychotherapist, I believe therapy is the best and most effective way to learn compassion, in particular in relation to ourselves. Psychotherapy is fundamentally a continuing lesson in how to be kinder, more forgiving and less hostile to ourselves and other people. It teaches us how to consider and understand each other's point of view and, importantly, how to then react in a compassionate way. Significantly, though, therapy teaches us to treat ourselves with compassion, to soften our inner critic, which is often the cruellest of critics, and to be less harsh towards ourselves when we perceive ourselves as failing. I have seen clients both struggle and succeed with the practice of compassion. Their stories remain confidential. All case studies contained in these pages are fiction. What I hope they illustrate is why childhood deficiencies and life experiences might make it more difficult for us to be compassionate. If you want to develop your compassion, I would urge you to find a therapist who can help you on your journey. But there are small things you can achieve working on your own. This book is, I believe, a great starting point.

As I was finishing writing I was confronted, out of nowhere, with compassion not as a force for good in our private lives, but as a source of argument and polemic in the public space.

'As an … American citizen, your compassion belongs first to your fellow citizens,' said J. D. Vance, Vice President of the United States, in January 2025, less than a fortnight after being sworn in. 'That doesn't mean you hate people from outside of your own borders. But there's this old-school – and I think it's a very Christian – concept … that you love your family, and then you love your neighbour, and then you love your community, and then you love your fellow citizens in your own country, and then, after that, you can focus and prioritize the rest of the world.'[3]

His positing of a *hierarchy* of compassion shocked many, especially coming from such a powerful figure in the new US administration and so high profile a convert to Catholicism. A few days later, the late Pope Francis entered the debate.

He did not mention the Vice President by name, nor did he use the explicit term 'compassion'. But his response did feel a bit like a slap down.

'Christian love is not a concentric expansion of interests that little by little extend to other persons and groups,' Pope Francis wrote in a letter to US bishops, citing the parable of the Good Samaritan for good measure.[4]

This book is not a treatise on the politics, philosophy or ethics of compassion. Its purpose is quite different. I hope it will be a starting point for you to think about the way you think and behave. This argument between two such influential figures only strengthened my conviction that this book is timely.

CHAPTER ONE

What Is Compassion?

Compassion is a complex word that is often misunderstood and misused. It is one of those words we all know, but rarely use in day-to-day conversation. We tend to use it as a stand-in for kindness, empathy or sympathy, but otherwise barely at all. In this chapter, I will define compassion and the qualities we need in order to practise it. I will also introduce the concept of self-compassion, an idea many people struggle with, and discuss evidence which suggests we can all learn to be more compassionate. Most importantly, this chapter will explain why compassion is good for us.

Defining Compassion

Compassion actually means much more than kindness or sympathy. There is an active part to it. The word derives from the Latin prefix com, *which means 'together', and the Latin root* passio, *which means 'to suffer'. Compassion literally means 'to suffer with or together'.*

The word has been in use in English since at least the fourteenth century, possibly earlier. The Oxford English Dictionary defines it as: 'The feeling or emotion, when a person is moved by the suffering or distress of another, and by the desire to relieve it.'

In simple terms, compassion is the desire to help someone who is suffering. It is recognizing and understanding that someone else is in difficulty and genuinely wanting to help them. It usually requires some courage because it forces us to look at other people's hurt and distress. And it always requires feeling moved enough to want to act. The crucial part of compassion is actually doing something – it is a motivational force. The action component of compassion distinguishes it from empathy, which is passive. Compassion is also very different to kindness. Acts of kindness, such as remembering someone's birthday, do not generally require an engagement with suffering, while compassion always does.

Compassion is part of what drives positive change in the world. It can inspire us to help people on a global scale. But it can also be really small. You are being compassionate when

'If you want others to be happy, practice compassion.

If you want to be happy, practice compassion.'

TENZIN GYATSO

The 14th Dalai Lama[6]

you donate to charity, volunteer for an organization or put a plaster on your child's cut knee. Compassion can be a call to a recently bereaved friend. Compassion is usually directed outwards, towards friends or strangers, but it can also be directed inwards to ourselves. So when you decide to stop beating yourself up for making a mistake at work, you are also showing compassion.

The last example is important, as it is an illustration of self-compassion. This is the turning inwards of compassion towards ourselves, our own problems and difficulties, however small, rather than ignoring or avoiding them. (Avoidance is always easier.) This essentially means treating ourselves in a less severe way when we are upset or struggling or when we perceive that we have failed in some part of our lives.

Self-compassion requires a bit of courage too, because it forces us to focus on what is upsetting us, rather than running away from it. It allows us to look at our problems in a compassionate way – which is always better than looking at our problems in an uncompassionate way.

Many people find the idea of self-compassion problematic. It is often seen as an indulgence, an attitude that allows us to excuse bad behaviour. But self-compassion often involves doing difficult things, such as having the courage to confront a self-defeating behaviour. In Western culture, in particular, self-compassion can be viewed as a 'soft' emotion, a barrier to self-improvement and ambition. We often believe that in order to succeed and do better we need to punish and criticize ourselves. In fact, it is crucial to be kind and forgiving.

Mistakes are an inevitable and unavoidable part of being human. When we view ourselves without compassion we may ruminate about our perceived failures or problems in such a way that erodes or destroys our happiness.

So compassion is many things: a moral force, an affective state, an emotional response, a human strength, a relational process and a path to greater awareness.

CASE STUDY: JOHN

John, 58, a retired solicitor, found it hard to get on with his elderly mother-in-law, Judith, who lived alone. She had been quite judgemental of him when he married her daughter, Veronica, and things had never really improved. She often made snide or supercilious comments about him, which he tried to ignore with some difficulty.

When his mother-in-law began to lose her memory, both he and Veronica worried about her declining health. John worried privately that his wife might ask if Judith could move in with them, something he didn't think he could tolerate. Some months later, Judith fell down the stairs and had to go to hospital for a broken arm. Soon, neighbours were calling, saying Judith needed help and they didn't think she was able to live alone any longer. John and Veronica eventually found an assisted living place for Judith near their home, where she could be monitored.

Soon, Judith was diagnosed with both pre-dementia and Parkinson's; Veronica struggled to accept her mother's mental state. The visits became distressing when Judith no longer remembered who she was. When Veronica told John this, he asked if it would help if he accompanied her on the visits. She said yes. John accompanied his wife every time she visited her mother, who died six months later, because he felt compassion not just for his wife, but also his mother-in-law.

Why Is Compassion Important?

It is difficult to overstate the importance of compassion. Research suggests that the giving and receiving of compassion can have major beneficial impacts on both our physical and mental well-being. If we cultivate and practise compassion towards others and ourselves, it can change the way we think, feel and behave – and even potentially alter how our bodies and brains work.

There is increasing evidence that behaving in a compassionate way stimulates parts of our minds and bodies which are associated with feelings of hope, calm and happiness. When we show compassion to others, or when we are self-compassionate, we actually make ourselves feel better. Some scientists call this the 'helper's high' or the 'giver's glow' because it is grounded in actual changes to our bodies, in particular a flood of hormones that make us feel good.

If we behave in a compassionate way towards ourselves, particularly when we are upset, self-critical or feeling like a failure, we might make ourselves feel less negative and more hopeful. Being self-compassionate helps us to bring our really difficult emotions like anger, disgust and fear more into balance, so that they don't dominate us and make us feel terrible. It is like being looked after by a compassionate mother when we are small. The compassionate mother wipes away our tears and makes us feel calm and happy again. This may sound a bit banal but there is a scientific basis for these claims which we will look at later.

Think of it this way: if you are focused on compassion, your mind will be organized in a compassionate way, rather than, say, an anxious, angry or critical way. You will be focused on being kind, helpful, understanding and empathetic to others. If we are focused on being compassionate to ourselves, our minds will be focused on being supportive, kind and caring to ourselves.

These ideas are not new. Compassion is an ancient concept found at the heart of all ethical and spiritual traditions. Almost every religion, from Hinduism to Islam, promotes the idea that compassion should be part of our lives.

Compassion is particularly revered in Buddhism. It is the second of the four divine abodes, or *brahmaviharas*, which are prized virtues. (The other three are loving-kindness, sympathetic joy and equanimity). Buddhists believe that cultivating compassion will help us to overcome self-centeredness, alleviate our own suffering and develop a sense of interconnectedness. 'I believe that at every level of society – familial, tribal, national and international – the key to a happier and more successful world is the growth of compassion. We do not need to become religious, nor do we need to believe in an ideology. All that is necessary is for each of us to develop our good human qualities. I try to treat whoever I meet as an old friend. This gives me a genuine feeling of happiness. It is the practice of compassion,' said the 14th Dalai Lama.[6]

Ancient Chinese traditions honour the figure of Kwan Yin who, by the ninth century, had become the main representation of compassion in China. According to legend, she tried so strenuously to alleviate the suffering of others that her head split into eleven pieces. The Hindu god Hanuman, a half-ape, half-human deity, is revered for using his powers in the service of others.

In the last twenty years, there has been mounting academic interest in compassion, not least because of increasing scientific-based evidence that its cultivation can have a major impact on our mental and physical health. Today there are many compassion-based organizations. Attempts are underway to cultivate compassion in schools. Companies are beginning to integrate concepts of compassion towards their employees, as well as in the way they conduct their business.

In 2000, Professor Paul Gilbert, a British clinical psychologist, created compassion-focused therapy, a psychotherapeutic approach that aims to help those who struggle in particular with self-criticism. Compassionate mind training was later developed to teach individuals, as well as staff, teams and organizations across a wide sector of professions, how compassion can bring a variety of mental and physical health benefits. You can read more about compassion-focused therapy and mind training later in the chapter.

As a psychotherapist, I often find that compassion is conspicuous by its absence. Clients may have grown up without much compassion around and, as a consequence, are not very good at being compassionate to themselves. They often have to learn how to grow their self-compassion muscle, and at the same time quieten the inner voice that is always punishing them for their failures.

The Components of Compassion

There is much discussion about the component parts of compassion. What emotional qualities does a person require in order to feel it? I am indebted to the work of Professor Paul Gilbert in formulating the following description of what constitutes compassion.[7] You will see that it requires substantial emotional work.

Non-judgement

When we are upset by something or someone, our first reaction can often be to judge and condemn. This blocks us from being compassionate. No one likes to see someone at the side of the street with an 'I am hungry' sign. Maybe they look unkempt, with a matted dog and a dirty sleeping bag. Sometimes it's easier to judge that unfortunate person and then walk away, rather than allow ourselves to be moved by their plight.

We often treat ourselves the same way. This means we condemn and judge ourselves for our perceived flaws and mistakes, even for the thoughts we have – the perhaps shameful or ugly things that are going on in our own mind. This makes us tend to either try to ignore them or to focus on them more intently, so that we get lost in a downward spiral.

Non-judgement means trying to step back from condemning ourselves. Learning to observe our thoughts, to see them for what they are, gives us a greater perspective. We become more aware of our thoughts and we can then learn not to act on them in an impulsive way.

Being Able to Tolerate Our Own Feelings

In order to show compassion, we have to be able to tolerate our own difficult feelings when confronted with something painful or difficult. Weeping after hearing from a friend who has suffered a personal tragedy is not compassion – unless you actually try to help them later. In fact, focusing on our own upset in the face of someone else's pain actually prevents us from feeling compassion.

This is also true of how we manage our feelings towards ourselves. We all have a variety of feelings. Sometimes, if these are difficult feelings like anger, disgust or sadness, we try to suppress them. Or we might do the opposite and wallow in them in a self-defeating fashion. Being compassionate means learning to be open and accepting of our own feelings. When we do so, we become more familiar with our feelings and less frightened of them. Part of being able to manage our own distress is also understanding that painful feelings will pass.

Sensitivity

Sensitivity is the ability to actually notice someone else's suffering in the first place. Some of us may not be aware that the friend we are talking to or spending time with is upset. We may be too busy thinking about ourselves to pick up on the fact that our friend is quiet, withdrawn or putting on a brave face.

Self-compassion means showing the same sensitivity to ourselves, and trying to tune in to what is distressing us.

Sympathy

You cannot feel compassion unless you feel sympathy. This means being aware, albeit without completely understanding, someone else's suffering. You feel sorry for their pain but from your own perspective. For example, if a friend loses their job, you won't necessarily feel their distress but you understand that your friend is sad. So there is some emotional distance with sympathy: you are not experiencing the pain yourself.

With self-compassion, having sympathy for ourselves allows us to get in touch with our own painful experiences.

Empathy

Perhaps empathy is the most important component of compassion. Empathy is the ability to understand what someone is feeling and to put ourselves metaphorically in their shoes. It involves feeling someone else's emotions from their perspective. To be empathetic is to have the imagination to see yourself in their place and understand what that person is going through. Empathy usually requires a bit of work on our part so that we can vicariously experience that person's feelings, perceptions or thoughts. The Oxford English Dictionary defines empathy as: 'the ability to understand and share the feelings of another.'

Self-empathy is similar – we have to think about what sits behind our thoughts or behaviour. Why are we drinking too much, for example. Is it to block something out?

The Motivation to Act

If you do not act, then you are not showing compassion. You have to want to have a go at being compassionate to others and to yourself. This means developing a willingness to look at things that may be difficult – rather than turning away. This is where courage is important, because being willing to engage with something problematic is usually not easy.

Other Components

Other academics might argue that compassion requires other qualities or conditions. They might say that the suffering that evokes our compassion needs to feel quite serious and to be the result of unfortunate circumstances. That is, it shouldn't be self-inflicted. It is important to add here that compassion is usually selfless, it doesn't require anything in return and it isn't motivated by self-interest. It is not transactional.

Can Compassion Be Taught?

Humans have the ability to intentionally choose to improve themselves. Just as we can go to the gym to increase the size of our biceps, so we can choose to improve our minds.

Compassion is not a fixed trait. There is now much academic research which suggests that compassion can be cultivated and strengthened with training and practice. Studies have also shown that compassion training can actually change the structure of the brain.

A 2013 study conducted by researchers at the University of Wisconsin-Madison established that adults could be trained to be more compassionate by using Buddhist meditation techniques.[8] (Buddhists have presumably known this for several thousand years.) Participants were asked to think of a time when someone they knew had suffered and were then

'Self-compassion is like a muscle. The more we practice
flexing it, especially when life doesn't go exactly according to
plan (a frequent scenario for most of us), the stronger and
more resilient our compassion muscle becomes.'

SHARON SALZBERG
Meditation teacher and author [9]

instructed to practise wishing that the suffering would be relieved. To help them focus on compassion they repeated phrases such as, 'May you be free from suffering' and 'May you have joy and ease.'

Participants practised with different categories of people, first starting with a loved one such as a friend or family member, someone whom they easily felt compassion for. Next, they practised compassion for themselves, and then a stranger. Finally, they practised compassion for someone they had been in conflict with, such as a colleague or flatmate. 'It's kind of like weight training,' Helen Weng, lead author of the study, said. 'Using this systematic approach, we found that people can actually build up their compassion 'muscle' and respond to others' suffering with care and a desire to help.'

The researchers also measured how much brain activity changed from the beginning to the end of the training, and found that the people who were the most altruistic after compassion training were the ones who showed the most neural changes.

In another study conducted by Mantelou and Karakasidou in 2017, it was found that even a short seven-minute intervention was enough to increase participants' feelings of closeness and connection and improve compassion and life satisfaction, when compared to those who received no compassion training.[10]

Compassion-focused Therapy & Training

All forms of psychotherapy are fundamentally focused on achieving the same goal, that is to help people to be less hostile and more forgiving towards themselves and others. Conventional psychotherapies, such as psychoanalysis or Cognitive Behavioural Therapy (CBT), have compassion at their core. A therapist always tries to create a compassionate relationship between themselves and the client and, in so doing, model a type of behaviour which may feel quite new. A therapist's aim is to actively engage with their client's suffering, so that the client may actively engage with their own. I have witnessed many clients learn and develop compassion and self-compassion.

Compassion-focused therapy is very specific in that it centres on teaching the skills and attributes of compassion. It aims to diminish problems related to feelings of shame, self-criticism and an inability to view oneself kindly. This type of therapy addresses issues varying from anxiety to eating and mood disorders. It has been used to treat children, teenagers and adults, and can be practised in individual or group sessions. Founder of compassion-focused therapy,

Professor Gilbert, states: 'One of its key concerns is to use compassionate mind training to help people develop and work with experiences of inner warmth, safeness and soothing, via compassion and self-compassion.'[11]

Compassion training uses exercises such as role-playing, visualization and meditation to help clients learn what compassion feels like and how to become better at practising it, both towards themselves and towards others. It also teaches clients how to recognize self-criticism and to develop techniques for defusing it when it arises. This may include visualizing their internal critic or identifying compassionate images to call to mind during moments of self-criticism. We will look in later chapters at techniques to help you be more compassionate to yourself and others.

Why Compassion Is Good For Us

One of the most significant themes of the novel A Christmas Carol *is Scrooge's extraordinary character transformation. When he learns kindness and compassion, he becomes a happier man, full of generosity and able to show love. He is no longer so isolated.*

The same thing is true for all of us. Being compassionate sets us free – it can liberate us from the prison cell of our negative emotions.

'Of notable relevance to mental health, compassion is not only
a process that builds positive relationships with others; it is
also a vital path to releasing the human mind from the
effects of harmful negative emotions.'

SHEILA WANG
Author[12]

In a fascinating experiment by Elizabeth Dunn, a professor of psychology at the University of British Columbia, a group of college students were given a sum of money. Half of them were then instructed to spend the money on themselves, while the other half were told to spend the money on other people, for example, by donating it to charity or buying a present for a friend. At the end of the study, the students who had spent money on others reported that they felt significantly happier than those who had spent money on themselves.[13]

The same phenomenon is true for infants. A study by Lara Aknin and colleagues at the same university showed that even toddlers as young as two exhibit greater happiness when giving treats to others than receiving treats themselves.[14] Many other studies have shown that compassion benefits not just our mental health, but also our physical health. In fact, some research suggests that it may speed up recovery from disease or even lengthen our lifespan.[15]

Here are some of the benefits of being compassionate:

Release From Harmful Negative Emotions

We all experience negative emotions; they are a normal part of human life. But there are times when they can weigh us down disproportionately. Learning to be more compassionate to others and to ourselves (like Scrooge) liberates us from the harmful thoughts we can have about ourselves and others.

Greater Sense of Contentment & Well-being

Being compassionate to others boosts our happiness. It is the equivalent of eating a piece of chocolate cake. In a 2006 study, Jorge Moll and his colleagues at the National Institutes of Health found that when people give to charities, it activates areas of our brain associated with pleasure, social connection and trust.[16] Scientists believe that compassionate acts release a flood of hormones, such as oxytocin and dopamine, which produce the positive feeling known as the 'helper's high', mentioned previously (see page 18).

Social Connection

When we are compassionate, we reach out to help others and this leads to greater social connectedness. This may well protect us from the health consequences of loneliness. A 2015 study of more than 2,000 people conducted by the University of Chicago found that extreme loneliness was twice as likely to cause death as obesity or high blood pressure.[17]

Being compassionate allows us to feel part of the wider world, part of a community, and this helps us, in turn, to feel supported. Volunteers live longer than non-volunteers, for example, but only those who volunteer for other-oriented reasons and not self-oriented reasons, as demonstrated by a study conducted in 2012.[18] Being compassionate towards our friends and partners also improves those relationships, allowing great intimacy and understanding.

Better Physical Health

Being compassionate improves our physical health. A study of elderly couples conducted in 2003 by Stephanie Brown of the University of Michigan found that people who provided practical help to friends, relatives or neighbours had a lower risk of dying over a five-year period than those who didn't.[19] This may be because being compassionate has been shown to lower our stress levels. High stress has long been associated with a range of health problems.

Improved Self-esteem

People who feel more connected to others have lower rates of anxiety and depression. Studies show that they also have higher self-esteem, are more trusting and cooperative and, as a consequence, others are more open to trusting and cooperating with them.[20]

COMPASSION IS CONTAGIOUS

In 2008, researchers from the Universities of California, San Diego and Harvard conducted an experiment which found that compassionate behaviour spreads from person to person.[21] When people benefit from kindness they 'pay it forward' by helping others who were not originally involved, and this creates a cascade of compassion.

What Is Self-compassion?

When we talk about compassion, it is usually in relation to others. Few people realize that we can (and should) also be compassionate towards ourselves. Practising self-compassion teaches us to handle life's challenges with a gentler, more forgiving attitude toward ourselves.

Self-compassion is the practice of being actively kind to ourselves, in response to feeling inadequate, having messed up or feeling ashamed. It is about treating ourselves in the same way we would treat a friend who is having a difficult time. We often don't realize how unkind we can be towards ourselves. How many times have you walked past a mirror and criticized the way you look? How often have you been out with friends and told yourself afterwards you weren't interesting or funny? Sometimes we aren't even aware of this critical inner voice because it is such a constant presence in our day-to-day lives.

'Talk to yourself the way you'd talk to someone you love.'

BRENÉ BROWN
Academic and author [22]

In the age of social media, self-judgement has become much worse. Everywhere we look, we see impossible standards of beauty, bodies we will never have, diets we can never follow, holidays we can't afford. Although we are all aware that social media is curated, we still somehow fall for it. We wish we were like other people and find ourselves failing.

This is true not just of external things like our appearance and the quality of our work, but also of our emotional, inner life. We criticize ourselves for our mistakes and failures. Why didn't we get that job? Why don't I get on with my sister? Why didn't I remember my friend's birthday? We all mess up; we wouldn't be human if we were perfect. Yet we often punish ourselves for not having the perfect family, for not being the perfect friend, the ideal parent, the best employee.

Being self-compassionate means becoming aware of this inner critic and taming it. Instead of always criticizing and judging ourselves, we try to be kind and caring towards ourselves, as we would a friend or someone in need.

CASE STUDY: MATTHEW

Matthew, 29, was very conflicted about his relationship with his parents. When he and his two sisters were younger, his parents had worked very hard in order to send their children to private schools. They had paid for all sorts of extra-curricular activities and made sure the children had great holidays, expensive birthday gifts and a beautiful home. Matthew was aware that his parents had constantly made him and his siblings conscious of the sacrifices they had made for them all. Even now as an adult, Matthew found that his parents were still reminding him of this, wanting something in return.

Matthew, who was married to a teacher, worked hard as a GP and was always exhausted by the end of the week. But his parents were constantly asking him and his wife to travel to see them at weekends, whether it was for family birthday parties or just a Sunday lunch. He always felt obliged to please them, to turn up and be sociable.

It took some time for Matthew to understand that he didn't need to say yes all the time, that he was allowed to say no; and that in saying no, he was actually giving himself a break from their demands, focusing on his own family and allowing himself time to rest.

The Three Components of Self-compassion

Dr Kristin Neff, an American academic and world-renowned expert on self-compassion, has identified three pillars to self-compassion:[23]

Self-kindness Instead of Self-judgement

Self-compassion means being kind towards ourselves when we feel bad or angry, rather than ignoring our own upset or punishing ourselves for our inadequacies. It means treating ourselves like a good friend would. This doesn't mean we don't acknowledge our shortcomings, it means we treat ourselves kindly when we fail.

Common Humanity Instead of Isolation

When we fail, we often think we are the only person in the world to have done so. This narrows our understanding and distorts reality. It can make us feel lonely and disconnected. When we are self-compassionate, we recognize that our suffering connects us rather than separates us from others. When we recognize we all mess up, it makes us treat ourselves with greater compassion.

Mindfulness Instead of Overidentification

We need to take a mindful approach to whatever is upsetting us. This means taking a balanced approach to it, neither taking it too seriously nor avoiding it. When we become over-identified with difficult thoughts and feelings we can often get swept away by them into a very negative space.

Why Self-compassion Is Good For Us

Just like compassion, self-compassion improves both our physical and mental well-being. People who are taught to be more self-compassionate tend to become less depressed and less anxious and are also less likely to suffer from excessive shame. They tend to be more optimistic and feel hope for the future. It's noted that they ruminate less and have lower levels of perfectionism and fear of failure. They tend to have a greater willingness to accept negative emotions and may be better able to cope with adversity.

Studies have shown that people who are self-compassionate generally have lower stress levels and better quality sleep, are more physically resilient and are less likely to suffer eating disorders or body-image problems.[24] They are also more likely to look after their physical health by eating well, exercising and avoiding harmful lifestyle choices like smoking.

Key Takeaways

- Compassion is how you feel when you see someone suffering and you feel moved to help them. Self-compassion is the practice of treating yourself with kindness, understanding and care during times of struggle, failure or when you are experiencing difficult emotions.
- Compassion has several components: non-judgement, being able to tolerate our own distress, sensitivity, sympathy, empathy and the motivation to act.
- Self compassion has three elements: self-kindness, common humanity and mindfulness.
- The skills of compassion and self-compassion can be taught.
- Compassion and self-compassion are good for our mental and physical well-being.

CHAPTER TWO

The Science Behind Compassion: Why We Are Wired to Care

It is tempting to believe that compassion is a modern attribute, a luxury we could only afford once we began to enjoy other benefits of civilization. Just as we are wealthier, healthier and better educated, so we must be more compassionate than our ancestors. Not true. In this chapter, I will illustrate how compassion was actually key to our survival as a species, allowing us to care for each other and create cooperative and successful groups. I will also explain the physiology of compassion: how it activates our brains and makes us feel happy, peaceful and even hopeful.

The Evolution of Compassion

It is too easy to mischaracterize early humans as brutal cavemen. Outdated stereotypes and historical misconceptions have helped to create an enduring image of our ancestors as violent and unintelligent.

The word 'Neanderthal' (referring to an extinct group of prehistoric humans who inhabited Europe and Western Asia between about 130,000 and 40,000 years ago) is often used as an insult, to signify someone who is crude, uncivilized and stupid. The use is so widespread in popular culture that even Joe Biden, former President of the United States, referred to the removal of mask-wearing during the COVID-19 pandemic as 'Neanderthal thinking'.

And yet, far from this brutish reputation, Neanderthals were actually intelligent humans. In fact, scientists now argue that they were also highly compassionate; indeed, this was one of the keys to their success as a species. Evidence suggests that even before Neanderthals, as long as three million years ago, our ancestor species may have looked after and helped each other to survive, even before they learned to speak. Though some of these species may have been physically unlike us, they were nonetheless capable of something very human.

Charles Darwin, along with many other biologists, argued that early humans were instinctually sympathetic. Darwin even went as far as to say that sympathy was an 'ever present instinct'. In *The Descent of Man* (1871), he wrote:

'Our capacity to feel compassion has ensured the survival and
thriving of our species over millennia.'

THE CENTER FOR COMPASSION AND ALTRUISM RESEARCH AND
EDUCATION, STANFORD UNIVERSITY SCHOOL OF MEDICINE[25]

'Those communities which included the greatest number of
the most sympathetic members would flourish best, and rear
the greatest number of offspring.'[26]

Why Did Early Humans Become Compassionate?

Evolutionary research suggests several reasons behind the
development of compassion in our ancestors.

The first is children. Like every mammal, early humans
needed to care for their offspring. If they didn't feed them,
respond to their needs, protect them, their children would
die. This would risk the survival of the group. Human babies
require unique levels of care over a sustained period of years.
The pressure to care for these vulnerable offspring, scientists
argue, gave rise to several adaptations:

* Powerful responses to a baby's distress
* The development of touching as a way to soothe
* Attachment-related behaviours between caregiver and
  offspring (wanting to be close to each other, distress when
  the caregiver leaves)

All of the above would have given rise to an experience we might call compassion, a trait designed to reduce any harm to vulnerable offspring.

Second, researchers believe that compassion evolved because it made us more attractive to potential mates. The more compassionate the partner, the more likely they were to devote more resources to offspring. This, in turn, was more likely to create the cooperative, caring communities that were so vital to the survival of children. It is thought that both females and males would have preferred mating with more compassionate individuals, a process that over time increased compassionate tendencies generally.

Third, many researchers believe that this mammalian caregiving system extended to encompass other members of the group, even non-family members and people who were ill or injured. Evolutionary theory suggests this was because helping others provided benefits to the individual themselves; it strengthened the group they belonged to and opened the doors to reciprocal helping. We needed capable, strong people in our social groups. Compassion enabled the kind of cooperation among strangers that advanced our species to where it is today.

What Does the Archaeology Say?

There is plenty of evidence to demonstrate how caring our ancestors were towards each other, as well as their infants. Fossil records indicate that early humans survived for many years after breaking bones or contracting serious diseases.

Archaeologists believe that other members of the group cared for them, attending to their injuries and ensuring they were fed, thereby ensuring they survived despite their helplessness or disability. There is also some evidence to suggest that groups cared for people who had suffered mental trauma.

Evidence: Shanidar 1

In 1957, the remains of a Neanderthal man who lived around 60,000 years ago were discovered in a cave in north-eastern Iraq. Archaeologists believe the man, who they named Shanidar 1, was aged between 40 and 50, the equivalent of about 80 years old today. He was found to have suffered several injuries, including a severe blow to the left side of his head, which may have caused partial blindness. He also had a withered right arm, possibly as a result of childhood disease. There is some evidence to suggest the arm may have been amputated, which, if true, demonstrates one of the earliest signs of surgery on a living individual. Shanidar 1 also had deformities in his lower legs and feet.

The condition of Shanidar 1 is important, scientists believe, because it suggests that Neanderthals cared for this vulnerable member of their group, allowing him to live much longer than he might have done if he had been left to his own devices. Someone so devastatingly injured could not have hunted or gathered his own food. He could not possibly have survived without care and sustenance. That he survived for years after his trauma was a testament to Neanderthal compassion and humanity.

Evidence: Windover Boy

In 1982 in Florida, archaeologists uncovered the remains of a boy who lived about 7,500 years ago. He had a severe spinal malformation known as spina bifida. His right shin ended in a gnarled knot of bone. His foot bones had withered away early in life.

Because the bone deformity would have taken several years to become so bad, researchers from Florida State University inferred the child must have been severely disabled for many years before he died, aged around 16. They believed the boy lived to this age because he was not abandoned and was cared for by his group. Their conclusion was that, contrary to popular stereotypes of prehistoric people, ' ... under some conditions, life 7,500 years ago included an ability and willingness to help and sustain the chronically ill and handicapped'.[27]

STAGES IN THE EVOLUTION OF COMPASSION

Archaeologists at the University of York, led by Dr Penny Spikins, have attempted to chart the development of compassion in early humans.[28] They believe there were several stages:

Six million years ago
This is when researchers believe the common ancestor of humans and chimpanzees experienced the first awakenings

of an empathy for others and motivation to help them. Compassion might have been displayed as a fleeting response to another's distress. This might have taken the form of an immediate gesture of comfort, such as a hug, or a very limited thinking through of an immediate problem such as moving obstacles in an individual's path.

Around 1.8 million years ago
This is when researchers believe compassion begins to be integrated with rational thought. There is evidence that pre-humans showed care towards the sick, pregnant women and those with young offspring. Researchers also suggest that evidence of burial practices demonstrate that pre-humans showed special treatment for their dead, that they mourned together and experienced grief together at the loss of a loved one, and that they wished to comfort each other over the loss.

In Europe between around 500,000 and 40,000 years ago
Around this time, human species such as Neanderthals developed much greater commitments to the welfare of others. This is illustrated by a dependence on hunting together and by the extended period of care shown to offspring. Researchers believe this demonstrated that Neanderthals experienced a shared emotional motivation to help each other. There is also archaeological evidence of the routine care of the injured or infirm over extended periods, such as Shanidar 1 (see page 41).

120,000 years ago
In modern humans, compassion was extended to strangers.

The Physiology of Compassion – Why It Makes Us Feel Good

We now know that throughout evolutionary history, humans have relied on compassion to survive. We also know that this mammalian caregiving system was designed to give rise to feelings of safety and calm, to relieve distress, to soothe those who were anxious and to protect them from harm.

Today, scientists are attempting to map the physiological basis of compassion to understand how it works in our minds and bodies. They believe that parts of our brain and our nervous system, as well as a range of hormones, are stimulated when we act in a compassionate way. All of these combine together to actually make us feel happy, peaceful, grounded and hopeful. Compassion actually feels pleasurable.

Dr Kelly McGonigal, a research psychologist and lecturer at Stanford University, formulated the following description of what happens in our minds and bodies when we are compassionate.[29]

Compassion is not that relaxing to begin with – because it always starts with a stress response. If we hear someone suffering or crying for help, for example, our nervous system is activated. The brain releases the stress hormone cortisol. This means that our heart rate increases and our pupils dilate. We sweat more. Our digestion processes decrease. Similarly, areas of our brain light up, including the amygdala, which detects threats, and the insula, which helps us to understand the pain of others. This is the body's 'fight or flight' response.

The fight or flight response is important because it is designed to pick up on threats quickly. It tends to promote unpleasant feelings in us, such as anger, anxiety or disgust, which are designed to make us take action to avoid the threat. That's good if you are crossing the road just as a car is coming. It's not so good if, as in our modern societies, our threat system is overstimulated because we are constantly in a state of stress about our work, our family, our parents, our mortgages.

The second stage of compassion balances this stress response with a calming experience. Our vagus nerve is activated, which actually slows our heart rate and breathing. (The vagus nerve is the main component of the parasympathetic nervous system, which oversees crucial bodily functions including control of mood, immune response and heart rate.) In fact everything about us slows down: our speech, our actions. We then tend to feel more centred and we can compose ourselves. This is the body's 'rest and digest' system.

Compassion depends on our ability to balance these two systems:

- A nervous system that experiences a stress response
- A parasympathetic system that calms us

In the final stage of compassion, a flood of hormones is released that motivates caregiving and social connection.

This includes oxytocin, the 'love hormone'. When you have higher levels of oxytocin, such as when you are experiencing compassion, you are better able to understand what other people are thinking and feeling. You are better able to be empathetic. Oxytocin also boosts the 'warm glow' we feel when we help others.

Oxytocin has an interesting side effect which is crucial in the experience of compassion: it inhibits the fear circuitry of the brain. This does several things: it helps our brain to read others, it increases our sense of courage and it inhibits our fear. It has also been found to enhance our motivation to support others.

Another important hormone is dopamine. This is a neurotransmitter which makes us feel great when we have a slice of chocolate cake or buy an expensive pair of shoes. Dopamine also gives us what Dr McGonigal calls the 'biology of hope'.[30] It tells us that if we act, something good will happen. This is important because even if we encounter something negative, dopamine will make us feel hopeful.

In other words, when we see suffering, we feel the stress of it first and then we empathize with it. This gives us the courage to respond with hope and kindness. When we do, our system rewards us and makes us feel good.

The Brain

Several brain regions play crucial roles in allowing us to feel compassion. Brain imaging has been able to detect which parts of the brain 'light up' when we are in a compassionate state, but the research is new and emerging. Also, many parts of the brain act together in complex ways. Here is a small sample of the areas of the brain that scientists believe are significant:

The Amygdala

The amygdala plays a central role in processing emotional information and is thought to be a core structure for empathy and compassion. Brain-imaging studies have shown that when participants view pictures of someone suffering, their amygdalae light up. Studies also show that compassion increases connectivity between the amygdala and the prefrontal cortex, which increases the likelihood that someone will help others, even at a personal cost. This is because this type of connectivity in the brain reduces reactivity to negative stimuli and decreases our anxiety. Interestingly, studies have shown that psychopaths have smaller amygdalae than the rest of the population.

The Anterior Cingulate Cortex

This part of the brain is central to processing emotional pain, particularly in others. It becomes active when we notice someone else's distress. This can then induce a form of discomfort which can motivate us to alleviate the suffering of others.

The Anterior Insula

This area of the brain is also involved in emotional processing. It helps us perceive and understand the emotional states of others. When we feel compassion, the anterior insula is often active, allowing us to share in another person's emotional experience.

The Ventral Striatum

This part of the brain is associated with feelings of pleasure: it creates the desire to seek out reward. When we make compassionate choices, the ventral striatum is activated in the same way as when we receive a personal reward.

Why Is the Science Important?

When we practise compassion during moments of stress or anxiety, our parasympathetic nervous system (rest and digest) kicks in and basically undoes the work of the sympathetic nervous system (fight or flight). It calms us down. It also encourages a feeling of safeness and security. It may also allow us to better understand our own mental state.

This is important because it means when we are compassionate to ourselves, we slow down, feel more grounded and have clearer minds – which means we will probably make better, more positive decisions.

Think back to the fight or flight response. This is the system that evolved in early humans as a way of dealing with life-threatening situations, such as an approaching hungry tiger. It protects us by putting us in a state of high alert, of stress, of thinking about danger and doing something about it. In our modern world, we don't need to worry about hungry tigers. Yet our threat system is still being activated. Today, we worry about modern problems such as how we look, can we afford to pay the mortgage, are our children thriving, do we have enough friends, have we put on weight. We engage in negative talk, in self-criticism and we overthink, all of which put us in a high-stress state. None of these require us to literally flee, run or hide.

When we constantly engage in self-criticism, are anxious, feel negative or angry, we not only activate our threat system, but we do so continuously, preventing our parasympathetic nervous system from kicking in. Consequently, we keep ourselves in this high stress-alert state. When our bodies are in this constant fight or flight response, we always feel on edge – ready to react to perceived threats when no real danger exists. This can lead to physical and mental health issues such as anxiety, depression, panic attacks, migraines, poor immune function and high blood pressure.

The key here is to understand that when we practise compassion, we activate the body's calming system. It's like a form of self-soothing. If we are able to be compassionate to ourselves when we are experiencing something difficult, we can make ourselves feel better. And the more we do it, the better we will feel. Many of us may have difficulty activating this self-soothing system because we may not have had the life experiences that give rise to it. This is what we will look at in the next chapter.

Key Takeaways

- Compassion evolved through the mammalian caregiving system and is part of what made humans thrive.
- Compassion has a physiological basis. Our brain, nervous system and a range of hormones are stimulated when we act in a compassionate way. They all combine to make us feel safe, grounded and hopeful.
- Modern life constantly activates our ancient 'fight or flight' response, which puts us in a high-stress state. This can lead to a variety of problems such as anxiety, panic attacks and high blood pressure.
- Practising compassion activates our body's calming para-sympathetic system, allowing us to self-soothe.

CHAPTER THREE

When & How Do We Learn to Be Compassionate?

If you want to develop compassion, it is important to understand how we learn it in the first place. Let's go back to the beginning, to childhood. Everything our parents and caregivers do, the way they behave, the way they manage their emotions, the way they discipline us, has a profound and lasting effect on our development and who we become. In an ideal environment, our parents treat us with compassion. But parenting is challenging, and parents don't always get it right. Sometimes, parents can – for all sorts of reasons – entirely or partially lack compassion. If children grow up in an environment where compassion is lacking, it can have a profound impact on the way they treat themselves and others.

Childhood

It may seem obvious, but when babies are born, they are unable to understand that someone may have a different mental experience to their own. They are profoundly egocentric. They also do not know they are separate from their caregivers.

This is why babies often respond to someone else's distress by becoming overwhelmingly distressed themselves. They think it's their distress. Studies have shown that, from a few months after birth, infants react to the pain of others as though it were happening to themselves.[31] On seeing another baby start to cry, they themselves begin to cry.

But there is an important moment in a child's development when they begin to understand that they are distinct from people around them. When children acquire the ability to differentiate themselves from others, they then begin to understand that other people may have different feelings to them.

Melanie Klein's Depressive Position

The depressive position is a developmental milestone in the first year of a baby's life when an infant realizes that its mother or caregiver can be both good and bad. Prior to this stage, the baby is only able to see its mother or caregiver in terms of wholly good or wholly bad. The baby cannot tolerate ambivalence, and instead exists in a world of extreme states of mind. In the depressive position, the child begins to be able to tolerate ambiguity and learns that good and bad exist within all of us.

This is important because it allows a child to broaden its tolerance, to understand that none of us is perfect, to see others as separate and to develop the capacity to feel concern about the welfare of the other. This is significant, of course, in terms of compassion. The theory was developed by Melanie Klein, a British psychoanalyst and one of the founding figures of psychoanalysis, who conducted pioneering work with children through observing their play.[32]

Jean Piaget's Theory of Cognitive Development

As children develop further, they begin to understand that different perspectives exist. When a child learns perspective, this is the first step on the journey towards learning what it might be like to stand in someone else's shoes – and to know and also care about what that feels like. This is one of the cornerstones of Jean Piaget's theory of cognitive development.[33] Piaget was a Swiss developmental psychologist who concluded that children understand other perspectives from around the age of eight. (Later studies have suggested that children younger than four can reliably adopt the perspective of others.) Children who understand that people have their own minds and therefore different perspectives are said to have developed a *theory of mind*.

This new sense of self and perspective is therefore key to the development of compassion. It allows a child to show concern for someone else who may be feeling quite differently to them. As children grow older, they gain the ability to experience empathy even when the other person is not physically present. By late childhood, children can empathize with another person's general plight – such as responding to a charity appeal on the television or when watching a nature documentary where a baby animal dies.

Parents As Teachers

Once children learn that others have separate feelings to their own, they then look and learn from their parents or caregivers. Most children live with their parents for eighteen years or so. It is an extraordinary length of time. Of all the animals on our planet, our long childhood is an extreme outlier. This environment operates all day, every day. It is an entire structure, a scaffolding, a way of life that has a profound effect on the way a child thinks and acts. Parents therefore play a crucial role in how a child develops compassion. The following sections look at the different ways parents can impact this development.

THE GOOD ENOUGH PARENT

It doesn't matter if parents fail sometimes; in fact it is helpful if children see that their parents aren't perfect. As the renowned British child psychoanalyst Donald Winnicott theorized, parents just need to be 'good enough'. The 'good enough mother' is a concept of a parent who isn't 'perfect' and who recognizes that it is impossible to respond to a young child's needs perfectly all the time.

Winnicott believed that it is essential that parents respond sensitively to a newborn's needs, sacrificing their sleep and time to allow a baby to thrive. But he also stated it is important, over time, to allow a young child to experience frustration and delay in having their needs met. This fosters a sense of the reality of the world in the child's mind, as well as a sense of independence.[34]

Identification & Internalization

Let's return to Ebenezer Scrooge. Why might he have become a cold-hearted and miserly adult? From a psychoanalytic point of view, it is easy to theorize that much of his character can be attributed to the environment in which he grew up and the messages and values he received.

Scrooge's mother died in childbirth and his father is portrayed as inhumane. He is sent away to boarding school and often left there at Christmas when his school friends return to their families. One can only try to imagine the loneliness, the sense of rejection, the grief and sadness of being at school over Christmas. How would a child cope with those profound feelings of rejection? One of Scrooge's only happy childhood memories is when his sister Fan, who later dies giving birth, comes to get him at Christmas, telling him their hard-hearted father had changed.

Later, Scrooge is rejected by his fiancée because of his love of money. A psychotherapist might speculate that it is perhaps no surprise that Scrooge transferred his feelings toward an inanimate object – money – rather than other human beings. Perhaps he thought money wouldn't let him down. Scrooge, who did not feel valued by his father, values money above all.

Scrooge received no love or compassion from his father. The two people who may have been capable of showing him love, his mother and sister Fan, are both dead. We can see how difficult it might have been for Scrooge to become a loving and compassionate person himself if his only parent cannot show love or compassion to him. He has no model, no one to learn from, no one to copy. Only his loveless father.

In psychoanalytic theory, Scrooge's adoption of his father's characteristics is what Sigmund Freud calls identification. This is an unconscious process in which children absorb and copy the traits of their parents. Identification plays a crucial role in the development of the personality of a child. This is fine if we have loving, nurturing parents – we will identify and adopt those qualities. It's not so good if we have a parent like Scrooge's father. Scrooge identified with his father's coldness, lack of humanity and cruelty.

When we identify with our parents, we also then internalize their values. Internalization is the process by which our parents' behaviour, morality, principles and moral codes are integrated into a child's sense of self and personality. Again, this is great if our parents are loving and kind, but not so much if you're Scrooge. He internalizes his father's moral code: he does not show love, closes his heart down, tells himself not to expect love and kindness and isolates himself from human contact. Scrooge grows up to be a man lacking in compassion not only to others but particularly towards himself.

Internalized Messages

When parents fail to show compassion in important areas of their children's lives, they can leave a void into which their unkind, unloving messages are stored instead. Scrooge didn't benefit from the warmth and good feelings that come from receiving compassion. His father's implicit and repeated message was: 'I don't care about you, I don't love you.'

When we don't receive compassionate messages as children (or as adults) we can develop all sorts of negative feelings about ourselves. We can feel unloved, unsupported, unimportant. We might have difficulty forming relationships, we might feel anxious, insecure and we might have problems regulating our emotions.

For example, if you grew up with a father who was constantly angry with you, you associate your father with fear and you grow up being fearful. You don't associate your father with warmth and kindness. You might think you don't deserve love and kindness. You might form relationships as an adult that are cold and unrewarding. Similarly, if you grew up with a mother who didn't have enough time for you, who was always busy, you might believe you don't deserve any attention or love or thought or care. You might feel worthless and insignificant. You might grow up and form relationships with people who make you feel small, insignificant, unloved.

Here are some other examples of parental behaviour which can affect young minds: favouritism, constant arguing, violence, criticism, bullying, abandonment, rejection and lying. Children usually develop defensive strategies to cope with these internalized messages and these can include: avoidance, suppression, hyper-independence, hypervigilance, perfectionism, self-criticism and neediness.

CASE STUDY: ANDREW

Andrew, 27, an only child, grew up with parents who were very busy. His father was a university professor and his mother ran a fashion business. She was often away organizing fashion shoots. One day Andrew went to work with a terrible cold. It was clear to his colleagues he should have stayed in bed. He was sneezing and coughing and had a sore throat.

When one of them told him to go home, he said 'I can't go home, there's nothing really wrong with me.' When his colleague told him that was patently untrue, Andrew recalled being told as a small child by his parents, 'There's nothing really wrong with you', whenever he was ill, or upset or just feeling sad.

If he felt ill or upset, his parents would mostly be dismissive of his illnesses or his feelings. Andrew interpreted his parents' 'There's nothing really wrong with you' quite literally: his illnesses or sadnesses were an inconvenience and there would be no sympathy from them. Psychoanalytically, one might theorize that Andrew identified with his parents, internalized their messages and behaviour and grew up treating himself and others in the same dismissive, uncompassionate way.

Andrew's internalized message was: you need to toughen up, don't be ill or sad, don't expect any sympathy from us. What did this message do? It dismissed Andrew's emotions and invalidated his feelings. How did Andrew react? He grew up ignoring physical and emotional pain.

EXERCISE: IDENTIFY NEGATIVE CHILDHOOD MESSAGES

Take a moment to think of ways in which your parents or caregivers may have given you negative, uncompassionate messages. I don't mean one-off messages, like a telling-off for eating all the biscuits without asking, but repeated narratives that tended to govern your childhood. Try to think about it now and write it down; it will be helpful for the next chapter. Perhaps it might look like this:

- You're so lazy, why can't you be more like your sister?
- I don't have time for this.
- You can't be tired.
- If you're naughty, I will punish you.
- You're always causing problems.
- You can't have that, we can't afford it, do you think we're made of money?
- You have to study the flute/violin/piano and I don't care if you don't enjoy it.
- Why aren't you more grateful? We work so hard for you.
- Go up to your room. I've had enough of you.

CASE STUDY: LUCIA

Lucia, 35, grew up the younger of two siblings, both of whom were pushed incredibly hard by their ambitious parents. At the age of 13, she was sent to a prestigious boarding school, which she hated. Lucia's parents had always referred to her older brother as 'the golden boy'. She could never match up. She felt like the black sheep, always disappointing her parents in comparison with her high-achieving brother.

Lucia's older brother left school to study at a top university and went on to work for an investment bank. Lucia, in an act of rebellion which upset her parents, didn't go to university and became a journalist.

Lucia found herself struggling at work after undergoing a fairly serious operation. She went back to work far too early and found herself in tears when colleagues asked how she was. She was perplexed by what she saw as this 'weakness'. Lucia was, unsurprisingly given her background, extremely competitive and had a punishing perfectionist streak. She wanted to be the best always, as a journalist, colleague, mother, wife. She had to be perfect at everything.

When Lucia began therapy, her analyst told her how exhausting it must be to burden herself throughout her life with this obsession with perfection. He told her she needed to learn how to be more compassionate towards herself, to stop punishing herself with the impossible standards her parents had placed on her. Perhaps she should have taken much more time off work after the operation. Lucia replied: 'I don't know how to be kind to myself.'

Lucia's internalized message was: why can't you be more like your brother. What did this message do? It created feelings of inadequacy and fostered competition, pitting siblings against each other. How did Lucia react? She grew up unable to feel happy in her own skin. She was constantly comparing herself to others and always finding herself failing. She felt she had to be perfect.

An Inner Voice

In these case studies, we can see that Andrew's and Lucia's parents failed to show compassion in important areas of their children's lives. When Andrew and Lucia required sympathy and kindness to help them when they were upset or not 'doing as well' as a sibling, their parents left a void, into which Andrew and Lucia poured two very negative messages.

These internalized messages become an inner voice. Freud called this voice the superego.

Superego

Freud believed there are three separate 'elements' to our minds: the id, the ego and the superego. These are not actual physical parts of the brain but rather hypothetical concepts as to how our minds work.

According to Freud, the id, the ego and the superego develop at different times and play different parts in our personalities. They all interact and together contribute to the behaviour of an individual.

- **The id:** This is the impulsive part of the mind that responds directly and immediately to basic urges, needs and desires. For example: 'I am starving, I am going to eat three doughnuts one after the other!'
- **The ego:** This deals with reality, ensuring that the id's basic impulses are controlled, reined in a little and expressed in acceptable ways. The ego is able to guide the id but it never has full control of it. For example: 'I will have one doughnut and then see if I am full.'
- **The superego:** This is the part of a person's mind that acts as a moral compass. It upholds a sense of right and wrong based on values that are initially learned from our parents. For example: 'I shouldn't eat a doughnut, I should have a green salad instead.'

Freud believed that the superego developed from the authority figures who surround us as children, mainly our parents (but also schoolteachers, for example) and that our superego functions as a reflection of their rules and regulations.

If a child has supportive, loving parents, they will probably develop a supportive and benign superego that helps them make moral choices which are sensible and reasonable. A healthy person usually has a superego that helps them to feel good about themselves and only punishes them by making them feel guilty for something they did that might have been wrong. In other words, a healthy superego is no different from a kind-but-firm parent: it has rules but it is also forgiving.

A particularly harsh superego will develop if a child has critical, harsh or emotionally absent parents. It will also develop if a child grows up with parents who are unable to be compassionate. When this occurs, the child will internalize this harsh, unforgiving, uncompassionate parent and they may become extremely hard on themselves, self-judging and self-critical. They may struggle to feel compassion. (Although conversely, children who have experienced harsh parents may actually become people-pleasers and be compassionate to a fault to others, but not to themselves.) They may also treat others in the same way. Look at Scrooge. In other words, an unhealthy superego is no different to a cold and punishing parent: it has too many harsh and unnecessary rules and is not forgiving or compassionate. In these cases, the superego becomes our 'inner critic'.

If we think back to the case studies of Andrew and Lucia, we can see their harsh superegos in action quite clearly. Andrew forced himself to get out of bed to go to work, even though he felt completely dreadful. What might his superego have been saying to him? Something similar to his parents? Stop feeling sorry for yourself. Your illness just annoys other people. Your boss will be cross with you if you don't turn up to work.

Lucia went back to work a few days after an operation, even though she was feeling fragile. What might her superego have been saying? You need to get better straight away, you can't be imperfect, you have to be better than you are, you have to be superwoman. Look at your brother – he can do anything.

Think about your own internalized messages. When you think of them, how do you feel? If your superego is a harsh one, it might sound and feel like this:

- It speaks in terms of the worst-case scenario and tries to convince you that the worst thing possible will happen. For example, I was so mean to my husband he will leave me.
- It generally speaks in terms of right and wrong or good and evil. For example, I am bad if I have a piece of chocolate cake; I am good if I have some lettuce. It is right to save all my money for my retirement; it is wrong to spend it on a holiday. It is wrong to buy that hardback book, I must wait six months for the paperback version. There is no nuance or grey area, everything is binary and extreme.

- When you think about these internalized messages, you feel overwhelmingly ashamed, guilty, reprimanded. For example, I made that mistake at work, everyone thinks I am stupid, I will get sacked, I had better resign.

Compassion can be the answer to this harsh superego. In the next chapters, we will look at how you can start to listen to this cruel inner voice and reflect on how to tame it – how to become more compassionate towards yourself.

Compassionate Parenting

Let's look at some examples of what compassionate parenting might look like, to give you an idea of how compassion does develop in children.

CASE STUDY: MARIANNE & JONATHAN

Marianne was struggling to adjust to life after divorcing from her husband. Recently, she had become worried about her teenage son, Jonathan, 15, who was particularly close to his father. He was suddenly not doing well at school and seemed to have lost a few friends. He had had a couple of detentions for not handing in homework.

Marianne was sharing custody with her ex-husband which meant Jonathan spent the weeks with her and every other weekend with his father. Until the divorce, Jonathan had seemed a relatively contented teenager. But after a call from Jonathan's school, telling her Jonathan was getting another detention, Marianne was reduced to tears. She was so angry that she shouted at Jonathan and told him to go and stay with his father permanently.

Jonathan rushed off and slammed the door to his bedroom, telling Marianne he hated her. Marianne immediately felt guilty and ashamed for shouting at Jonathan. She texted a girlfriend for advice and then called Jonathan's father. After a while she was able to calm down. She then went to speak to Jonathan, in a calm and compassionate way, and was able to have a conversation with him about what he was feeling and why he was getting into trouble at school.

Marianne knew that Jonathan hadn't simply become 'bad' or 'naughty' but that he was expressing his sadness, frustration, grief and anger at his parents' divorce. Jonathan was able to tell his mother, through his tears: 'I just get really upset when I have to swap homes, leave you or Dad, I just want things to be like they were before.' Marianne showed compassion towards her son. She didn't punish him for not handing in his homework (although she made it clear that homework was non-negotiable).

She instead saw that he was suffering, and she reached out to talk to him. Together they were able to work out that perhaps Jonathan needed to spend more time with his father.

CASE STUDY: WILLIAM & TOM

William felt he had never really got over the death of his mother when he was 18. At the age of 40, he was married with two children and worked as a television producer. His life was very busy. William had begun to worry about his son, aged 6, who was becoming more and more envious of his little sister, aged nearly 4. His son, Tom, had screamed at him one morning: 'I wish Jemima had never been born!' William was incredibly upset about this and shouted at Tom for being nasty about his little sister.

William later felt annoyed with himself for shouting at his son, after discussing with friends how 'normal' it was for children to be jealous of their younger siblings, who they perceive may be getting more attention than them or depriving them of parental time and love. One of his friends told him how positive it was that Tom was able to freely express his negative feelings for his sister. This, of course, made William think of all the feelings he didn't express – particularly about the death of his mother. After his mother died, his father had removed all photographs of her from the house and they never talked about her again.

William was able to see that he might be repeating his own father's mistakes in not allowing his children to express quite natural feelings. He realized he needed to talk to Tom about his feelings for Jemima, rather than shouting at him, and see what emerged. He and his wife also thought more carefully about the time they spent with Tom and Jemima and how they might make it more equitable.

The Outcome of Compassionate Parenting

What happens in scenarios like these two case studies, where compassionate parenting is shown? The two children, Jonathan and Tom, learn that they are not 'bad' for feeling the way they do. They learn that their parents will be compassionate towards them when they feel upset, sad or if they have done something 'wrong'. They do not feel they have to hide their feelings, or be ashamed of them. They learn that they are loved in all their complexity, for their flaws as well as their strengths. They learn that love will not be withheld.

Attachment Theory

Attachment theory is important because, along with many other psychoanalytic concepts, it helps form an understanding of how we behave as adults. Attachment theory is also connected to compassion. Many researchers believe that if a child experiences a difficult or problematic attachment to their parents, it may well lead to difficulties with compassion.

Attachment theory is based on the work of the British psychoanalyst John Bowlby. Bowlby believed that the relationship between children and their parents sets the stage for how they relate to themselves and others for the rest of their lives. He called this connection between caregivers and babies 'attachment'.[35] The central theme of the theory is that parents who are available and responsive to their child's needs allow them to develop a sense of security. The infant learns that the caregiver is dependable, which creates a secure base for the child to then explore the world.

Researchers believe that children who feel safe, secure and loved in this way are much more likely to have the capacity to be sympathetic and compassionate to others.

If a child does not have her needs consistently met, if she is neglected in times of upset and if her parents are cold and unavailable, she will grow up with an insecure attachment, where she finds it hard to trust others and the world does not feel secure. Children with insecure attachments grow up into adults who have low self-worth and are untrusting.

Unsurprisingly, children with a secure attachment are much more likely to be able to feel empathy and compassion as adults. Children who grow up in an environment where they don't feel secure or safe are much less likely to be able to show compassion for others, or indeed themselves.

CASE STUDY: JIMMY (INSECURE ATTACHMENT)

Jimmy, 28, a musician, had left his boyfriend of three years and was feeling increasingly isolated and unhappy. He wasn't sure why he had left his boyfriend, as they had been 'fairly happy' together. After several months, Jimmy told his therapist that he often felt a sense of self-loathing, which was worrying him more and more. He found himself constantly criticizing himself and telling himself off for minor indiscretions. Jimmy was a freelance musician and, although a prestigious studio had offered him a job, he had turned it down. His income was therefore unstable and he did not feel part of an organization.

Jimmy had an insecure attachment style. He had grown up with a single mother, who held down several jobs and was often physically violent towards him. His mother frequently punished him for reasons he couldn't understand or justify. Jimmy never knew his father. This is a good example of an insecure attachment style, which is characterized by a lack of both trust and a secure base.

People with an insecure style may behave in anxious, ambivalent or unpredictable ways. Jimmy refused a stable job, left his boyfriend without really knowing why and isolated himself. We can also see Jimmy's inability to be compassionate towards himself – he was constantly criticizing himself, punishing himself and making himself feel 'bad', just like his mother had done.

CASE STUDY: MICHAEL (SECURE ATTACHMENT)

Michael, 31, a private tutor, wanted to leave his marriage. His wife, who didn't work because of a minor disability, had been unfaithful with an ex-lover. Michael had tried hard in his marriage, had supported his wife financially, but felt he could no longer trust her. Michael felt bad for wanting to leave his marriage. He felt he had failed in some way and was embarrassed and ashamed to tell his friends and in particular his widowed father, who had enjoyed a long and very successful marriage.

When he was finally able to tell his father, he received a compassionate response. Not only did Michael's father suggest his son seek therapy to help him through what was likely to be a stressful few years, he also – despite his advanced years – helped Michael move out of the marital home, recognizing that the move would be very emotional and difficult for his son.

Michael behaved honorably towards his wife during the divorce process, making sure that she would have enough financial stability to live on her own, even though this meant reduced circumstances for himself.

This is a good example of generational compassion. Michael's father behaved compassionately towards his son during his divorce, doing what he could to alleviate his upset. Michael, in turn, although with very mixed feelings, treated his wife with compassion during the divorce, ensuring she came out of the legal process with a fair financial settlement.

Michael had a secure attachment style. He wasn't afraid to leave a bad marriage; he knew he deserved better and that he could start again. Someone with an insecure attachment may well have stayed in a bad marriage, lacking the confidence and security to leave, believing they didn't deserve better.

Key Takeaways

- We learn compassion in childhood through our parents and caregivers, and also through authority figures like teachers.
- We internalize messages from these figures and they become part of our everyday thinking, our superego or our inner critic.
- Sometimes, if we have parents lacking in compassion, our superego becomes harsh and cruel and we treat ourselves and others in an unkind and uncaring way. We fail to treat others and ourselves with compassion.
- If we grew up with parents who were unable to love us in a consistent, kind and supportive manner, we develop an insecure attachment style as adults. We may feel anxious, untrusting, insecure and fearful and have difficulty feeling compassion towards ourselves.

CHAPTER FOUR

How Can We Learn to Be More Compassionate?

You should now have a better idea of what compassion is and how it can be helpful when you or others are struggling. Maybe you have learnt several things about yourself and compassion. Perhaps you have reflected on whether you might have grown up without particularly compassionate parents or caregivers and now find it challenging to treat yourself and others in a thoughtful, non-judgemental and caring way. Maybe you have thought about your inner critic too and what it sounds like. Perhaps you have established that this inner critic can sometimes be a bully that makes you feel anxious and self-critical – making it hard for you to show compassion. In this chapter, we'll consider how you might start to be more compassionate.

Starting With Our Thoughts

Becoming more compassionate doesn't necessarily require years of therapy. (I would always recommend therapy, though, as the most effective route to accessing our thoughts, behaviours and patterns, many of which are unconscious.) One of the key skills in learning to be compassionate both to ourselves and to others is to pay attention to what is going on in our minds. This isn't always as easy as it sounds.

Remember that we have all sorts of thoughts and feelings going on inside our heads that we have internalized from childhood, many of which we may be quite unconscious of, but which nevertheless profoundly influence the way we behave every day.

Freud's Conscious & Unconscious

Freud theorized a model of the mind in which there are two distinct levels: a conscious and an unconscious. The unconscious part of our minds contains thoughts, desires and memories that are not accessible to our day-to-day awareness, but which still have a fundamental effect on the way we behave. In fact, Freud believed that the unconscious has a fundamental influence over daily life. The conscious part of our minds, on the other hand, contains the thoughts and feelings which we are aware of at any given moment.

It is important to hold this in mind because accessing our unconscious is usually only possible with the help of a psychotherapist or analyst. However, there are ways in which we can begin to learn to be more aware of our unconscious thoughts, feelings and behaviours so that they do not govern us without us realizing.

Old Brain/New Brain

There are many ways of conceptualizing how our minds work. Some therapists, particularly in compassion-focused therapy, like to use another concept called old brain/new brain to explain how our minds work.

Many researchers theorize that we have two different types of brain. We have an 'old brain' that evolved many millions of years ago that does very similar things to other animals' brains, such as alerting us to hungry tigers. Remember the stress response, the 'fight or flight' response we discussed in Chapter 2? This is the 'old brain' at work.

However, about a million years ago, our 'new brain' evolved, which allowed us to plan, imagine, analyse and make judgements. Our new brain allowed us to consider the past and the future. It also allowed us the ability to think about thinking. These new brain abilities, while fantastic for human progress, can cause us all sorts of problems, like overthinking, ruminating or imagining worst-case scenarios. Whereas an animal will forget about the hungry tiger once it has disappeared, we humans might use our new brain to carry on thinking and worrying about it. We might create terrible scenarios in our heads about tigers. So we then re-trigger our fight or flight response.

The more we trigger the old brain into fight or flight, the more our new brain becomes stimulated and starts to see more danger in more situations. Our bodies fill up with stress hormones and we lose touch with the rational part of our brain. It's hard for us to think in a calm and considered way.

For example, imagine you are driving to the supermarket when another driver cuts you up and you have to brake suddenly. You quickly become furious and sound your horn and even silently swear at the other driver. This is our old brain working, reacting to an actual threat – there was some danger involved. If we aren't very good at calming ourselves down, we may still be thinking about this driver half an hour later. We may still be stressed and angry about it. We may go home and be irritated with our partner. This is the new brain ruminating and overthinking and keeping us in a high-stress state.

Fortunately, we have the ability to be mindful – which means stepping back from our thoughts and observing them. By being mindful of our thoughts, we can actively engage our new brain into thinking more rationally. We can then try to redirect our thoughts in a compassionate way and tell ourselves to put the irritating driver out of our mind.

'Our life is what our thoughts make it.'

MARCUS AURELIUS (121–180 CE)
Roman emperor[36]

Becoming Aware of Our Thoughts

How can we become more aware of our thoughts? It sounds simple but it can be so difficult. If we don't know what our thoughts are or what our inner critic is telling us, then they control us.

If we want to tame our inner critic and reframe our self-critical voice so that we can be kinder to ourselves and others, we first have to become aware of our thoughts. This is where *thinking about thinking* comes in. Some therapists call this mindfulness, but I find mindfulness is a tricky word that often makes people grimace. Thinking about thinking, or developing awareness of our thoughts is literally that – the process of becoming aware of our thoughts.

This is a crucial skill for compassion because it helps us to stand back, be self-aware, perhaps even be non-judgemental when responding to both our own suffering and the suffering of others. It helps us to become more observant of ourselves, our reactions and our feelings so that we don't run off into an unhelpful state of panic, criticism, anger or anxiety. It allows us to make better decisions, to maybe change the direction of our thinking or attention. Gradually, we can train ourselves to notice when our negative thoughts are taking over and realize that thoughts are simply thoughts – they do not necessarily have to control us.

For example, imagine you are expecting a member of your family home from a work trip abroad. You call them but they don't answer. You call again, puzzled. Some of us would be rational and remain calm and sensible. If we felt worried, we might try to be self-compassionate and tell ourselves to try not to panic or let our thoughts run away with us to imagine some terrible catastrophe. Some of us, who are less capable of being rational, for all sorts of reasons that we have looked at earlier in this book, might start panicking. The panicking mind, now in a state of high stress, runs away into a negative place, imagining plane crashes or train derailments, even a terrorist attack.

If we can learn to be more aware of what we are thinking, of where our mind is taking us, we might be able to stop ourselves from rushing recklessly into this upsetting place. Wouldn't that be less exhausting?

Why Is Self-awareness Important in Compassion?

Self-awareness is crucial because it allows us to be aware of both our own feelings and those of others. We may otherwise miss signs of distress in others or fail to acknowledge our own pain. It also helps us to feel centred and calm, rather than getting caught up in negative thoughts that make us feel stressed and unable to think positively or constructively.

Significantly, self-awareness helps us be less judgemental, more accepting and more understanding of ourselves and others, which opens the door to compassion. It also helps us to regulate our emotional responses. Self-awareness can create a more balanced emotional base, so we avoid feeling overwhelmed by difficult things that happen to us or others. It helps us to avoid reacting impulsively or in an uncontrolled, unconsidered way when faced with difficult emotions or situations.

Learning to become aware of our thoughts isn't easy and can be frustrating. In time, though, we might be able to begin to notice patterns of behaviour that influence our daily lives, relationships and our professional selves. This awareness will allow us to respond to everyday situations in a more rational and compassionate way, rather than reacting out of habit or impulse.

Attention

How we direct our attention is crucial. Attention is defined as the act or state of applying the mind to something. When something negative happens, it is possible to train ourselves to direct our attention and thoughts to something helpful and positive.

HOW TO BE MORE AWARE OF YOUR THOUGHTS

- **Observe your thoughts.** Stand back and listen to what your thoughts are. Are you concentrating on the task at hand or are you ruminating on some past upset or future scenario?
- **Be aware of your inner critic.** Try to observe your inner critic, which we discussed in Chapter 3. Can you recognize it and then dismiss it?
- **Give your thoughts a name.** When you feel tense about a meeting with your boss, tell yourself that this is anxiety about the meeting. Nothing more.
- **Try to remain in the present.**
- **Practise meditation.** This helps you become more aware of your thoughts as they come in and out of your mind.
- **Rest your mind.** This is like taking a breather when you are at the gym. It could be something simple like going for a walk or listening to music.
- **Become more aware of your body.** If you have a pain in your shoulder, is it because you feel tense about a meeting? If so, do you really need to feel so worried about it? If you really are worried about it, is there anything you can do about it?
- **Take a break from social media.**
- **Prioritize sleep.** Lack of sleep can lead to a range of mental-health problems.
- **Learn a mindfulness practice.** Mindfulness practices involve intentionally focusing our attention on the present moment, without judgement, using techniques like mindful breathing or walking.
- **Start working with a therapist.**

For example, if a friend who is usually reliable cancels a long-awaited lunch at the last minute, you can choose how to manage your disappointment and irritation. You can get angry with your friend, have a row and make the situation worse. Or you can be understanding, forgive them for having to cancel and rearrange the lunch date. Now, suddenly you have a spare couple of hours. What will you do?

In this example, you either direct your attention to the fact that your friend has let you down and get upset – or you remind yourself how she is usually reliable and that something must have cropped up that was unavoidable. You try not to judge. You give her a break. You then go shopping for some new pyjamas in your spare two hours. Which is likely to make you feel better?

CASE STUDY: MELANIE

Melanie was a successful writer who was crippled by insecurity in her romantic relationships. She often picked unsuitable men who were untrustworthy or dishonest and treated her badly. The relationships didn't last. Melanie had grown up with a musician father who was often abroad on concert tours and a mother who she described as 'unavailable'.

While in therapy, Melanie fell in love with a writer who was significantly older than her and often away at literary festivals, tours or speaking engagements. They soon moved in together. Melanie frequently told her therapist how unreliable her boyfriend was, and that she feared he was quite selfish. But this seemed at odds with other stories she told about him. When the therapist dug deeper, it became clear that Melanie's boyfriend was actually caring, communicative and loving. It was just that Melanie tended to direct her attention to negative thoughts about his behaviour. When she told her therapist about a time when she was ill with the norovirus, she said that her boyfriend had told her afterwards how difficult it was for him to look after her. 'How selfish is that', she said. 'Do you think I should leave him?'

The therapist wondered if Melanie could instead direct her attention to the fact that her boyfriend uncomplainingly looked after her for three days while she was suffering. Saying that looking after her had been a struggle was simply a statement of fact, not evidence of selfishness. This was the first step in Melanie's journey towards reframing how she directed her attention and thoughts about her boyfriend and, indeed, others.

Reasoning & Thinking

Negative thinking drags us down. It makes us anxious, miserable and depressed. We can instead try to think and reason in a more productive way. When we are compassionate, we deliberately choose to refocus our thinking in ways that are more likely to make us feel secure, happy and stable.

'There is nothing either good or bad, but thinking makes it so ... '

WILLIAM SHAKESPEARE (1564–1616)
Playwright and poet[37]

For example, imagine that a friend who is usually always in touch suddenly goes quiet and you don't hear from them for a few weeks. Compassionate thinking and reasoning would allow you to reason that they are just busy, preoccupied or possibly ill. Uncompassionate thinking would take you down the negative route of believing they don't like you anymore or ruminating that you have done something to upset them. Before you know it, you feel upset and anxious.

Thinking things through can be difficult because it requires us to look at difficult feelings. Often, we don't like to consider what we are thinking, for all sorts of reasons. Thoughts can be painful, shameful, upsetting, negative. For example, you might not want to think about how annoyed you are with your out-of-touch friend, because it makes you feel insecure, unlikeable, mean or infantile. You might not want to dwell on a stupid mistake you made at work because it makes you feel ashamed. Sometimes we just want to get rid of these feelings. We certainly don't want to talk about them. This is when we might reach for a packet of biscuits or alcohol or anything that might distract us.

Learning to be compassionate towards ourselves and others can help us to get a better grip on our thoughts.

Rather than running away from our thoughts, we can deliberately look at them, with the intention of not letting them control or dominate us. Compassionate thinking involves learning to become more aware of how negative emotions can direct our thoughts. We can then try to make a deliberate choice to consider what is helpful. Compassionate thinking allows us to stand back from our emotional reactions and choose a more constructive path.

CASE STUDY: JOE

Joe had a difficult childhood with absent parents and found it hard to feel secure in relationships. He often found himself leaving partners after a year or two, having convinced himself that they didn't really love him or weren't properly committed to him. He wanted his current relationship to be different. But he found his girlfriend's behaviour challenging. She didn't tell him she loved him that much, she was totally absorbed by her work and she often left all the social arrangements to him. He felt this was evidence that she didn't really care for him.

Joe came to understand that his childhood with absent parents, who were always away working, had affected his feelings of self-worth. He had internalized their absence as him not being worthy of their presence. He didn't feel deserving or worthy of love. Because he felt so worthless, he was always looking for evidence of this in his relationships.

Joe often didn't reason or think in a compassionate way. Rather he leapt to negative, threatening or anxiety-inducing thoughts. When his girlfriend started talking about moving to France, he immediately assumed she meant on her own, without him. This wasn't true – but Joe had leapt to a conclusion, formed in childhood, that his girlfriend didn't want him. He often thought this way, even when his girlfriend did something quite ordinary, like not pick up a call.

Joe tried to reframe his thinking, so that he didn't see the world through this negative lens of being unloved and unworthy. He tried to adopt a more compassionate view of himself and his girlfriend. Why would she tell him she wanted to move to France, unless she meant both of them? He knew she wasn't cruel, or unhappy in the relationship. When she didn't answer a call, perhaps it was because she was in a meeting, not because she didn't love him.

Behaviour

The way we behave in the world has a huge impact on the way we feel. Compassion is about working out how to alleviate our own or someone else's distress.

This can be in the form of doing pleasant things, like recognizing we need to walk around the park after a difficult meeting with our boss, but it can also mean doing difficult things like saying no to someone who takes advantage of us, or choosing to intervene when we notice someone is struggling. Behaving in a compassionate way, particularly

HOW TO THINK & REASON IN A COMPASSIONATE WAY

- Be aware of your own thoughts and emotions, recognizing when you might be starting down a negative path of criticism, judgement or shame.
- Ask yourself the following:
  - Is this thinking helpful to me?
  - Would I think like this if I weren't upset?
  - Would I teach a child or friend to think like this?
  - If not, how would I like to teach them to think about these things?
- Try not to judge others or yourself.
- Be more tolerant and accepting of yourself and others and be aware that everyone makes mistakes.
- Use compassionate, helpful, encouraging and supportive language when thinking about yourself and others.
- Remember that everyone has their own struggles.
- Ask questions – how can you help?
- Consider how you would like to be treated.
- Stay present and avoid defensiveness.
- Acknowledge your limits: compassionate reasoning doesn't require you to solve everyone's problems.
- Set healthy boundaries: compassion doesn't mean tolerating harmful behaviour or letting others take advantage of you.
- Consider the bigger picture: compassionate reasoning often requires thinking beyond immediate reactions and focusing on the long-term well-being of all parties involved.

HOW TO BEHAVE MORE COMPASSIONATELY

- Do one compassionate thing every day, for yourself and/or for someone else, even if you don't feel like it.
- Practise gratitude. At the end of the day, try to remember kindnesses that you gave or received.
- Be forgiving of yourself and others.
- Practise small acts of kindness, like opening a door for someone.
- Listen to what people say to you and ask them questions.
- Do one small pleasurable thing for yourself each day, whether it's buying yourself a coffee or calling a friend.
- Volunteer.
- Try to see yourself as part of a connected world in which cooperation and kindness result in better outcomes.
- Silently wish other people well, wishing them happiness and freedom from suffering.

towards ourselves, is not just about being nice. For example, it can be quite challenging to enquire after a colleague who is clearly performing really badly at work, or to suggest to your grumpy teenager who just shouted at you that maybe she would like a cup of tea and a chat. It is often much easier to just ignore them and hope their problems will disappear.

CASE STUDY: SARA

Sara led an incredibly busy life as a corporate lawyer as well as being a stepmother to her husband's two sons. She also volunteered for the Samaritans and helped out at her local church. She had lots of friends and was always organizing dinner parties and Sunday lunches. She had one particular friend, though, who was often critical of her and she couldn't understand why. She was particularly generous to this friend, who was single and often said she felt lonely. But Sara found that, however kind she was, however many Sunday lunches she invited her to in order to help her feel less lonely, the friend never felt it was enough.

Sara grew up with parents who did not tell her they loved her. Her mother suffered from depression and her father, who she said 'was not a family man', was always bad-tempered and angry. She felt so unwanted that she turned herself inside out trying to please her parents. Sara was soon able to see that she was also turning herself inside out to please her friend. Sara wasn't able to stop – she just kept doing more and more. After talking this through for several months, Sara was able to see herself more compassionately and accept that she was enough just as she was. It was quite a revelation. Instead of feeling she had to do more and more to please her friend, she was now comfortable doing less.

Key Takeaways

- Freud believed we have a conscious and unconscious. Our unconscious has a profound effect on the way we live our daily lives.
- We have old brains and new brains. Our new brains cause us all sorts of problems, like overthinking, ruminating or imagining worst-case scenarios. This triggers our fight or flight response which makes us feel stressed and anxious.
- To be more compassionate to ourselves and others, we need to learn to be aware of our thoughts so that they don't dominate us and make us feel anxious and stressed when we encounter problems in our lives.
- Learning to be mindful of our thoughts is the first step to becoming more aware of how our minds are working. Mindfulness is the practice of paying attention to our thoughts in the present.
- We can then try to think, reason and behave in a more compassionate way towards ourselves and others.

CHAPTER FIVE

How Can We Be More Compassionate to Ourselves?

In a world that encourages comparisons, competition, self-criticism and perfectionism, it can often be easy to neglect our own well-being. While we may be willing to show compassion to others, when it comes to ourselves we can be our own worst critics, judges and jailers. How can we embrace a more compassionate approach towards ourselves? As we discussed in Chapter 1, there are three core components to self-compassion: self-kindness, common humanity and mindfulness. In this chapter, after establishing how self-compassionate we currently are, we'll return to these components and look at some practical ways to cultivate self-compassion.

EXERCISE: HOW SELF-COMPASSIONATE ARE YOU?

This exercise helps establish how self-compassionate you are. The following is an adapted version of the work of Dr Kristin Neff, a pioneer in the field of self-compassion research, who developed the first Self-Compassion Scale.[38] This was the first tool of its kind specifically developed to measure self-compassion. You can do the full version online: (self-compassion.org/self-compassion-test).

The following statements describe how you act towards yourself in difficult times. Read each statement carefully and then indicate how often you behave in the stated manner on a scale of 1 to 5, with 1 being almost never, and 5 being almost always.

1. I try to be understanding and patient towards those aspects of my personality I don't like.
2. When something painful happens, I try to take a balanced view of the situation.
3. I try to see my failings as part of the human condition.
4. When I am going through a very hard time, I give myself the caring and tenderness I need.
5. When something upsets me, I try to keep my emotions in balance.
6. When I feel inadequate in some way, I try to remind myself that feelings of inadequacy are shared by most people.

For the next six statements, use the following scale (note that the scale is reversed from the previous set of statements): 1 is almost always, 5 is almost never.

1. When I fail at something important to me, I become consumed by feelings of inadequacy.
2. When I am feeling down, I tend to feel that most other people are probably happier than I am.
3. When I fail at something that is important to me, I tend to feel alone in my failure.
4. When I am feeling down, I tend to obsess and fixate on everything that is wrong.
5. I am disapproving and judgemental about my own flaws and inadequacies.
6. I am intolerant towards those aspects of my personality I don't like.

Now, add up all your answers, then divide the total by 12 to find your average (mean) self-compassion score.

As a rough guide to understand your score:

• A score of 1 to 2.5 indicates you are low in self-compassion.
• A score of 2.5 to 3.5 indicates you are moderate in self-compassion.
• A score of 3.5 to 5.0 means you are high in self-compassion.

Self-kindness Not Self-judgement

To be compassionate towards ourselves, we have to actively engage with our problems. More often than not, though, we get caught up in a storm of self-judgement that prevents us from doing this. Many of us have no idea how unkind we are to ourselves on a minute-by-minute basis.

Think of all the people you know who constantly put themselves down. Nine times out of ten, we will automatically beat ourselves up when we make a mistake. This is so pervasive in our wider society that we almost don't notice the phenomenon. The problem with judging ourselves is that it creates stress and anxiety and stops us from thinking clearly, constructively or helpfully, which is the opposite of self-compassion.

Read the following questions and see how many of them you answer yes to:

- When you last walked past a mirror, did you criticize an aspect of your appearance?
- When you last ate, did you later tell yourself off for eating too much, not eating the 'right' thing, having dessert?
- When you last met up with friends, did you compare yourself to them unfavourably?
- When you last bought something for yourself, did you feel bad afterwards for spending the money?

- When you last came home from work, did you look back at the day and judge yourself for not doing a piece of work as well as you would have liked?
- When you last told off your child or got annoyed with your partner/parent/sibling, did you think you were a bad parent/partner/sibling afterwards?
- When you last went to a dinner party, did you criticize yourself for not making sparkling conversation?

Many of us will have answered yes to all of these questions. This exercise is a very simple way to illustrate the incessant nature of our self-critical voice. One of the hardest things to do is to catch ourselves at it. Noting when we are criticizing ourselves is the first step to greater self-compassion.

This is not to say that we shouldn't criticize ourselves or that we should let ourselves 'get away' with bad behaviour. Often people think self-compassion will make us complacent and too forgiving of ourselves when we mess up. I will examine this later in this chapter.

Today, self-criticism is particularly problematic thanks to social media, which forces us to constantly compare, judge and condemn ourselves. We are flooded with images of perfection: bikini bodies, happy families, incredible holidays, beautiful homes, extraordinary weddings. It is extremely difficult not to get caught up in this world of perfection, even when we understand, rationally, that these images are digitally altered, filtered, shot at a certain angle, saturated with false colour, to the point that they bear no resemblance to reality. Even though we know rationally that no one has a face without flaws or a body without a bit of a wobble, we are very good at convincing ourselves otherwise.

Identifying & Transforming Your Self-critical Voice

Identifying our inner critic can be hard. It is usually doing its work when we suddenly, without much explanation, slip into a bad mood, become upset or angry, afraid or overwhelmed, or even quite child-like. More often than not, you will find, if you listen hard enough, it is our inner critic which is pulling us down, making us feel upset.

The exercise on pages 100-01 can help you to identify and reframe your self-critical voice. Here are some other ways of transforming your inner critic:

- **Give your inner critic a name.** Try to create a distance between yourself and your inner critic by giving it a name or face.
- **Practise self-gratitude.** Write down one thing you are grateful for about yourself each day.
- **Keep a self-gratitude journal.** Look at it often to remind yourself of your strengths and achievements.
- **Use affirmations.** Write them down. Stick them on your bathroom mirror. Repeat them when you are feeling low.
- **Examine the evidence.** If your inner critic tells you that you are worthless, examine the evidence – do you have a partner, friends, family who value you? Could you speak

to them to get feedback? When you hear your inner critic talking, stop what you are doing and redirect your mind by doing something you enjoy, whether it's going for a walk, listening to a podcast or doing some baking.

- **Practise mindfulness, meditation or deep breathing.** This will help you stay present and distance yourself from negative thoughts.

CASE STUDY: STEPHEN

Stephen, 60, had grown up in a wealthy family with three siblings and a busy father who was strict and withdrawn. His father was a leading cardiologist who was often away in the States lecturing if he wasn't operating. His mother had died when the children were young and Stephen's father appeared to have withdrawn into a state of grief covered up by constant work and travel. The four children were expected to 'just get on with it' most of the time.

Stephen, who worked for a charity, was struggling with writing a report for the board of trustees. He was finding it increasingly difficult to concentrate. Stephen repeatedly criticized himself, telling himself he was stupid for not being able to finish the report: it was pretty straightforward, anyone could do it, what was wrong with him? Why couldn't he just get on with it? This hostile inner dialogue crippled Stephen, leaving him unable to write for hours. The more behind he became, the more he would punish himself.

With some help from his therapist, Stephen tried to reframe this hostile inner critic and learn how not to talk

EXERCISE: REFRAME YOUR SELF-CRITICAL VOICE

Think of a time when you felt anxious or nervous. It could be when you were at a party and had to talk to someone new, or when you were taking a driving test or an exam. Then think of what you said to yourself at the time. Write it down. Try to be as accurate as possible. What critical words did you use? Did the voice remind you of anyone from your past? A parent or teacher? Familiarize yourself with the sound and texture of this voice.

For example:

- That person at the party won't want to talk to me, I don't have anything interesting to say, I'm inferior and dull, I won't be able to entertain them.
- I'll fail this exam. I didn't study hard enough. Part of me is really lazy and just isn't as good as everyone else.
- I made such a stupid mistake at work, everyone will think I'm useless and will be talking about me behind my back, wondering why I even have a job here.

Now try to actively reframe what you said to yourself. Try to soften the words, speak as if you were speaking to a friend.

to himself like his father did. He thought about things that made him feel good, like running, baking bread and listening to history podcasts. Stephen decided that the next time his inner critic started beating him up, he would stop what he was doing and indulge in something else, something that absorbed his mind completely and made him happy.

Ask yourself, would you use these words to someone you loved? Use warm and supportive vocabulary, even if it feels embarrassing or ridiculous.

For example:

- I understand you feel shy and awkward but that person has never met you before so how do you know they won't want to talk to you? You're an interesting person with lots to say. Maybe they're shy too? It's not your job to entertain them!
- I've studied really hard for this exam and I'm ready for it. I'll do my best and that'll be enough, that's all I can do. I shouldn't compare myself to everyone else.
- I did make a mistake, but everyone makes mistakes and I know my boss will be understanding. This is a useful lesson and I'll make sure I don't mess up again.

You may want to take this further and actually speak to your inner voice. Even if it sounds a bit silly, it might be worth a try. You could say something along the lines of: 'I'm not listening to you. There's no evidence or facts to back up what you're saying. Please be quiet. You're not a very constructive voice and I'm closing you down.'

The next time he found himself stuck in the middle of his report, feeling guilty and ashamed, he went for a walk while listening to a podcast. He found he was able to return home in a better state of mind, which freed his thoughts from their negative spiral, allowing him to make some progress on the report.

'The very definition of being 'human' means that one is mortal, vulnerable and imperfect. Therefore, self-compassion involves recognizing that suffering and personal inadequacy is part of the shared human experience – something that we all go through rather than being something that happens to 'me' alone.'

KRISTIN NEFF
Academic and author[39]

Common Humanity Not Isolation

Everyone fails. There is no normal. Famous people are just like us – they do not lead perfect lives. People in the public eye, from politicians to film stars, have problems just like ours: concerns about their children, their appearance (you aren't allowed to age if you are famous), their aging parents, their next job ...

If we do badly at something, it can help if we try to think that everyone messes up. If we immediately tell ourselves we are the only ones who ever fail this way, our negative feelings will multiply. We will feel isolated and alone. We can end up in quite a dark space, and this becomes a vicious circle. This negative self-talk is often quite unconscious. We live in a world that celebrates success, while failure is ignored. So our thought processes are programmed against failure.

If we tell ourselves that everyone makes mistakes, we can help ourselves to feel less alone, less miserable about our failures and less guilty and ashamed. Just as with self-kindness, read the following sentences and see how many of them feel familiar to you:

- Why wasn't I invited to that party, that's so mean. Why don't they like me? What's wrong with me?
- I did really badly in that interview. I'll never get a job.
- My son didn't make it into the football team, that's not fair, he's going to feel so alone and upset.
- How come I don't have a partner, everyone else does.
- I just made a terrible mistake at work, I'm the only one in my team who messes up, my boss must be so disappointed in me.
- I totally forgot I was having coffee with my friend and now she'll judge me and not ask me for coffee again.

These are the kinds of thoughts we have when we forget that everyone messes up, gets upset, feels like a failure.

The exercise on page 105 can encourage self-compassion by reminding you that everyone makes mistakes and you are not alone. Here are some other ways to remind yourself of our common humanity:

Meditation
Sit somewhere quiet and gather your thoughts. Maybe close your eyes. Think of someone you know, but not that well,

perhaps a work colleague or even a celebrity. Then think of something that has made you feel bad recently – maybe you had an argument with a friend, or you told a lie in order to get out of something you should have attended. Then ask yourself, does my colleague or that celebrity ever feel the same way I do? Do they ever argue with their friends? Do they ever lie? Ask yourself the question several times, and feel how your bad feelings about yourself lift when you think that others have messed up like you.

Journal
Try to write down things that make you feel bad about yourself, ashamed, isolated, guilty. It could be a time when you shouted at your child and made them cry because you were stressed, or you criticized your partner for something minor. Then do some research online or survey your friends. Have your friends or other people online done the same? How did it make them feel? Did they feel the same as you? If they did, can you sense that this makes you feel slightly better?

Mantra
Think of a form of words that could help you, such as, 'Everyone feels bad/ashamed/stupid/guilty sometimes, even [insert the name of a celebrity or well-known person you admire].' Stick it on your bathroom mirror or fridge, or somewhere else where you can see it everyday.

EXERCISE: EVERYONE STRUGGLES

The following is adapted from an exercise created by Dr Kristin Neff.[40] It is designed to remind you of the three components of self-compassion when you are feeling anxious. Think of something that is upsetting you in your life. It could be work-related or something about a friendship or relationship. Visualize the situation clearly. What is the setting? What is happening? Who is saying what to whom? Can you feel discomfort in your body as you bring this difficulty to mind?

Now try saying to yourself: 'This is a moment of suffering.' Then say to yourself: 'Suffering is part of life.' Other options include:

- I am not alone.
- Everyone experiences this, just like me.
- This is how it feels when people struggle in this way.

Now try saying to yourself: 'May I be kind to myself.' Other options include:

- May I accept myself as I am.
- May I begin to accept myself as I am.
- May I forgive myself.
- May I be strong.
- May I be patient.

Take a moment to reflect on how the experience of this exercise was for you. Did you find the reminder of common humanity helpful? Some of the language above may feel a bit silly at first. Sometimes it takes a bit of time to find the language that works for you and feels authentic.

CASE STUDY: LIVIA

Livia was a personal tutor who came to therapy because she was suffering from anxiety. She was a reserved young woman who had grown up with diplomat parents who moved country every few years. Livia had found the constant moving incredibly destabilizing and the need to make new friends stressful and exhausting. Her parents were unsympathetic, seeing it as a 'wonderful opportunity' for Livia to see the world.

Livia had one student she particularly liked because she reminded her a bit of herself at the same age – very shy and reserved but clever. She had been teaching her for several years but her time with the student was now coming to an end because she was going to university. Livia was worried about the final class and how she would feel. Normally she signed off her students with no trouble at all. After the final class, Livia found herself crying uncontrollably and could not understand why. 'I felt so silly and ashamed,' she said. When she told her girlfriend after the class, her girlfriend said: 'But nobody died.' Livia promptly shut up and dried her tears and said no more.

With some help from her therapist, Livia was able to understand that it wasn't strange that she was upset, that it was not unusual to feel grief and sadness at the ending of a relationship like the one she had with her student. We often feel a sense of grief when a relationship comes to an end, even if it is not romantic. It could be any relationship that is meaningful to us.

'I've lived through some terrible things in my life, some of which actually happened.'

MARK TWAIN (1835–1910)

Author[41]

Livia started crying again and told her therapist it was a great relief to be told she was 'allowed' to cry, because this is what most people did.

Mindfulness Not Overidentification

We talked about mindfulness, or 'thinking about thinking' as I prefer to call it, in Chapter 4. But it is worth looking at it again. This kind of awareness of our thoughts is at the centre of self-compassion.

If we break mindfulness down to its essence, it can be summed up as paying attention to our thoughts in the present moment. This means that we try to stay in the present moment, not the past or the future (which do not exist). We are fully aware of where we are and what we are doing. Being mindful allows us to focus on what is within our control and to let go of what is not. It allows us to concentrate on the present and to stop worrying about the future.

When we aren't mindful, our thoughts take flight and before we know it we can be obsessing about something negative that happened in the past or something frightening about the future.

Being aware of our thoughts is important in self-compassion because it prevents us from becoming 'over-identified' with difficult thoughts and feelings, so that we aren't swept away by them. It also means letting go of resistance to whatever problem life throws at you. For example, if you find six people ahead of you in the coffee queue and you are late for work, you might get angry and frustrated. You might be annoyed that the people ahead of you will make you late for work. Becoming aware of your thoughts in this moment might allow you to say to yourself that it isn't surprising there is a queue, everyone wants to get a coffee before work and that this is just the way it is. It won't necessarily make your time in the queue pleasant, but it may help you to be calmer and more at peace while you wait.

MINDFULNESS EXERCISES

If you look online, you will find hundreds of resources that will teach you how to be mindful. Here are a few of my favourites.

Be more aware of your environment: Next time you feel stressed about something, go for a walk, take time to look at the trees in your street or notice the smell of the fresh coffee in a cafe, rather than letting your mind run away and become overwhelmed with all the things you have to do at work that day.

Be more aware of your body: Next time you feel a pain in your shoulder or a tightening in your chest, ask yourself what is happening. Are you anxious about something? If so, what? Try to bring it to mind and understand what it is that's bothering you. Do you have guests coming to stay and the house is a mess? Try to bring your thoughts to the present moment, what you are doing in the present, reminding yourself that the future will take care of itself. I often find the Mark Twain quote on page 107 really helpful – and it makes me laugh.

Focus on your breathing: When you have negative thoughts, try to sit down, take a deep breath and close your eyes. Focus on your breath as you inhale and exhale. Sitting and breathing for even just a minute can help. A favourite doctor of mine taught me a useful rhyme to recite when feeling stressed: 'When in doubt, breathe out.' You can also try the breathing exercise in Chapter 6 (page 130).

CASE STUDY: LAWRENCE

Lawrence, 24, was extremely upset when his girlfriend of two years left him. He had been happy in the relationship and hadn't seen that she was becoming increasingly distant and unavailable. Lawrence found he could not stop himself from following his ex-girlfriend on social media, trying to figure out if she was dating someone new, who she was on holiday with, whether she had moved jobs. Lawrence would spend hours going down rabbit holes. He worried this obsessive behaviour was becoming unhealthy.

One of Lawrence's problems was that he had too much time on his hands. His job as a part-time accountant was fairly relaxed so he had time to indulge in his obsession. He hated himself for it but couldn't stop.

Lawrence was aware of what he was doing in the moment – it wasn't unconscious. He thought about the ways he might stop his mind from spinning out of control and causing him pain. He looked at some mindfulness and journalling exercises online – ways of bringing his mind back to the present moment. After buying a nice leatherbound notebook, Lawrence started a journal and found himself writing notes to himself, like 'Stay off Instagram, it's unhealthy' or simply 'STOP', to remind himself not to go down the social media rabbit hole. Lawrence was able to bring himself back into the present with his journal, and to stop his mind running away with him to painful spiralling behaviours.

What Self-Compassion Is Not

Many people worry that self-compassion is a form of indulgence, the opposite of the British stiff upper lip. They think it is selfish or a form of victimhood or weakness. Some people find the idea of being kind to ourselves just plain wrong. Surely we have to be tough with ourselves in order to become stronger?

Often, we think we need to be hard on ourselves in order to achieve success. Being kind to ourselves when we perceive we have failed often seems to stand at odds with a society that rewards us for our professional and social accomplishments. But there is now much research which shows that self-compassion is a far more effective force for personal motivation than self-punishment.

Juliana Breines and Serena Chen from the University of California at Berkeley conducted several experiments in 2012 examining whether being self-compassionate after making a mistake can increase one's motivation to self-improve.[42] The researchers showed that participants who were more self-compassionate demonstrated greater motivation to change personal weaknesses following an initial failure than those who were less self-compassionate.

Self-compassion, far from being a way to evade personal accountability, actually strengthens it. At first this may seem paradoxical. Dr Kristin Neff has formulated the following responses to misconceptions about self-compassion:[43]

It Isn't Self-pity

Many people fear self-compassion is a form of self-pity. Neff argues that it is an antidote to feeling sorry for oneself because it reminds us that everyone makes mistakes. This makes us less self-obsessed and less focused on our own flaws.

It Isn't Weak

Being self-compassionate is actually a source of strength and resilience. Being supportive and kind towards ourselves, rather than beating ourselves up all the time, makes us stronger in the long run. Research shows that self-compassionate people are better able to cope with tough situations. Self-compassion is also about having the courage to face our problems, rather than running away from them. That isn't weak.

It Isn't Selfish

Some people ask, if we turn compassion inwards, isn't that a form of self-centredness? Actually if we face up to our own flaws and problems in a compassionate way, we are much more likely to do the same to others. In fact, it can enhance our ability to care for others.

It Isn't Lazy

Many people believe being critical and harsh on ourselves compels us to succeed. So, it follows, self-compassion must be a form of laziness. In fact, it is a proactive way of dealing with difficulties, mistakes and challenges. It doesn't mean avoiding responsibility.

It Isn't Letting Ourselves Off the Hook

Some people fear that being kind to ourselves means we allow ourselves to get away with bad behaviour. In fact, self-compassion allows us the freedom to admit to mistakes we have made, rather than blame others. Research shows that self-compassionate people take greater personal responsibility for their actions and are more likely to apologize if they have offended someone.

Key Takeaways

- We can all find practical ways to be more self-compassionate.
- We can identify and transform our inner critic through techniques such as journaling, meditation and affirmations.
- If we come to understand that everyone messes up, that this is part of being human, we can start to learn to be kinder to ourselves.
- Being aware of our thoughts can keep our minds in the present and help us be more compassionate to ourselves.
- Self-compassion is not weakness or indulgence; in fact, it is an act of strength.

CHAPTER SIX

Self-Compassion in Relationships & at Work

Relationships are hard. This is particularly true of romantic relationships. Intimacy means opening ourselves up to love, being vulnerable, learning to trust, being forgiving and letting go of perfection. Being more self-compassionate in our relationships benefits both ourselves and our partners. It makes us more trusting, more forgiving and better at resolving arguments. Being more self-compassionate can also benefit us at work, where we can be particularly self-critical and harsh towards ourselves. Research shows that if we can learn to be kinder to ourselves in our workplace, we often perform better.

Strengthening Romantic Relationships

Often we expect our marriages or partnerships to live up to an ideal, where our partner is attuned to our every need, want and desire. Think of all those scenes in your head: perfect couples with perfect children in a perfect house with a perfect sex life.

We all know this is fantasy and that all partnerships are messy, sometimes boring, often difficult and usually challenging. No partner can fulfil our every need. If we haven't had the parenting we need as children, we often look to our partners to fill the hole that was left. But our partners can't be our parents, and hoping they will can only lead to disappointment, arguments and unhappiness.

Learning to be more compassionate to ourselves can help us in our romantic relationships. Research shows that self-compassionate people generally have happier and more satisfying partnerships. A joint German study carried out in 2024 by the universities of Otto Friedrich in Bamberg and Martin Luther in Halle-Wittenberg found that being more forgiving of one's own shortcomings in a romantic relationship can lead to greater happiness among couples.[44] Lead author Dr Robert Korner said: 'We found that one's ability to react compassionately to one's own inadequacies, suffering and pain in the relationship benefits both members of the couple. In this way, an actor's self-compassion not only improves their own happiness, but also their partner's.'

'We all marry our unfinished business ... We are thrown back
into the soup of our relational traumas from childhood.'

TERRY REAL

Licensed Independent Clinical Social Worker (LICSW), Author of *Us:
Getting Past You & Me to Build a More Loving Relationship*[45]

Forgiveness & Understanding

Self-compassion generally makes us more forgiving of
ourselves. When we upset our partner, we don't immediately
punish ourselves. (This doesn't mean we allow ourselves
to get away with bad behaviour towards our partner.) Self-
compassion allows us to look at our mistakes with an element
of kindness, so that we are then able to pluck up the courage
to say sorry.

For example, we might come home from a bad day at work,
blame our partner and start a row that might allow us to get
rid of those bad work vibes. Self-compassion might allow us
to look at what we have done and to understand we were
using our partner to evacuate some bad feelings, which isn't
good. We might then think, everyone does this from time to
time, it's rubbish of me, I shouldn't do it, I will try not to do it
again, now I need to apologize.

There is evidence that if we overly punish ourselves for
being rude or unkind to our partners, it creates a downward
spiral where we get locked into a negative space where self-
blame and inadequacy actually prevent us from apologizing.

Self-compassion can also work in the opposite direction, when our partner upsets us. Rather than shouting at them, slamming a door and walking away in tears, we can be kind to ourselves. We can ask ourselves if we are upset, why are we upset? Have we gone to a dark place because our partner came home from work in a bad mood and was less than charming, or is it because his or her bad mood reminds us of our father or mother and we feel infantile and scared? Obviously we *can* just be upset about the bad mood, but more often than not when we overreact it is because we are reliving some past interaction from our childhood. Was your father always in a bad mood? Did you have to tread on eggshells so as 'not to disturb Daddy'? Did your mother not listen to you when you were upset?

Asking ourselves what might be causing us to overreact to our partner's bad mood might just lead us to a better understanding of ourselves, and therefore of our partner also. Similarly, if we think of the common humanity theme discussed in Chapter 5 (page 102), we can try to tell ourselves that everyone has a partner who is a bit rude sometimes, so we should give them a break. Your thoughts might go something like this: 'Okay my partner upset me and I'm annoyed, but they probably just had a bad day and are taking it out on me. I could escalate this or just make them a cup of tea. Then later, when they're calmer, I'll tell them not to take stuff out on me.' Being self-compassionate allows us to be more compassionate to our partners, forgiving them more easily and understanding they may have had a bad day and need some help from us.

Trust, Acceptance & Kindness

When people feel safe to express their needs and feelings, bad as well as good, trust increases. If we are self-compassionate, we tend to be less defensive and therefore more trusting of ourselves and others. This allows for greater acceptance of our partner, flaws and all. In a 2012 study by Neff and Beretvas, people who were compassionate to themselves were described as being significantly more accepting of their partners, and also granted them more autonomy.[46] Because self-compassionate people accept themselves as imperfect human beings, they may be more inclined to accept their partner's limitations. Similarly, given that self-compassionate individuals are kind and caring toward themselves, they may be more inclined to give partners the freedom they want to make themselves happy.

People who are more self-compassionate are more likely to be kind to their partners. This is because when we are self-compassionate, we are better at regulating our emotions and tend not to use our partners as punchbags. It also makes us more patient and empathetic with our partners, less resentful and more resilient to whatever problems our relationship throws at us.

Equal Relationships

Self-compassionate people are better able to balance their own needs with their partner's. They generally don't form co-dependent relationships where there is a mismatch of needs. This tends to lead to more equal relationships where no one can take on a controlling attitude to the other. When we have healthy self-esteem, we usually have better intimate relationships because we are more accepting of ourselves and others. Our healthy sense of self-worth means we don't accept unhealthy relationships or breadcrumbs. If a partner treats us badly, we ask for better behaviour, knowing we are worth it.

CASE STUDY: SORAYA

Soraya, 40, a musician, was unsure she wanted to continue in her marriage. She felt huge frustration with her husband, Tom, who came from a very British stiff-upper-lip family. Soraya and her husband had a whirlwind romance, married very quickly and had two sons. It was only when Soraya was emerging from the depths of rearing small children that she began to find fault in Tom. 'He doesn't do emotion', she said. 'When I'm upset he just closes up! It's not that difficult, all he has to do is give me a hug! What's wrong with him?'

With some help from a therapist, Soraya tried to foster a more self-compassionate view of herself when she was upset. Why did she expect Tom to make her better? Why was it his responsibility? Was it always his fault? What was she upset about, really? Soraya had grown up with a younger sister who had suffered leukaemia at the age of three; as a result, all of her parents' attention had been diverted to her sister. When Soraya got upset as a child, her parents had been unable to look after her in a consistent way and she had been forced to find ways to soothe herself. In her marriage now, she was looking to Tom to parent her.

Soraya thought about the ways she could be kinder to herself in those moments of upset, rather than demanding something of Tom. Could she soothe herself? She began to find ways to talk to herself. Rather than saying, 'I'm so upset, I need Tom to fix this', she tried, 'It's okay to feel this way right now. Let's not run away into a dark place, I can try to handle it.' Soraya also taught herself to pause when she was upset and try to focus on the ways Tom demonstrated his love towards her. Maybe not in the way she wanted, such as a hug, but in the way he knew how, like cooking dinner for her or bringing her a cup of tea in the morning.

It's Not About the Dishwasher

When we are upset or arguing with our partner, we can find ourselves in turmoil. Trying to figure out what caused the argument, so that it doesn't happen again, is a self-compassionate way to approach disagreements.

Think of the last time you felt upset with your partner. Try to remember what it was that triggered it. Was it something minor like the dishwasher not being emptied, or something more significant? Try to remember how you felt at the time. Anger, sadness, frustration? What did you do in that moment? Did you immediately get angry and start shouting? If so, why? Did it lead to a row? What did your partner say to you? Did they get defensive and start shouting back?

Let's imagine your partner borrowed and then lost something important to you, for example, an expensive scarf. The scene may have gone something like this:

You: 'How could you have lost my favourite scarf! I've had that for ages, it was a gift from my best friend! I can't believe you did that. You just don't care about me. This just shows how you feel about me that you can't take care of my things. You don't value my things or me ...'

Them: 'Don't shout at me, I didn't mean to lose it, it was a mistake. I am really sorry!'

You: 'No you aren't sorry! You just don't care about my things, you are so disrespectful and uncaring. I wish I had a more caring partner.'

Them: 'That's such a mean thing to say, I am not disrespectful and uncaring. How dare you say that. That is just typical of you, you are so reactive and rude ...'

And so the argument spirals into a slanging match with no kindness, compassion or generosity, just name-calling and anger and a state of warfare.

Let's go back to that moment when you discovered the scarf was lost. You probably felt anger, disappointment, irritation and upset. But if you take a moment, you may discover that the anger and disappointment are not really about the scarf or even your partner. Your partner, in all likelihood, didn't intend to lose your scarf, and even if they did, it probably wasn't about any lack of respect for you but because they are forgetful or didn't realize its significance or they were busy and distracted.

HOW TO BE MORE SELF-COMPASSIONATE IN RELATIONSHIPS

- Be aware of your thoughts and feelings, where they are coming from and what they might mean.
- If you upset your partner, apologize, but don't get caught up in a negative spiral of blame or even shame.
- Be open and honest with your partner about your needs, desires and hopes.
- If your partner upsets you, let them know in an adult, non-confrontational way.
- Give yourself space from your partner. Cultivate friends and colleagues.
- Speak to yourself in a positive, hopeful way. Negative self-talk can erode your confidence and contribute to feelings of inadequacy or unworthiness.
- Don't compare your relationship with those of others.
- Acknowledge small wins, like getting through a particular challenge together.

Your anger and disappointment is in all likelihood related to an unmet childhood need. Arguments between couples are rarely about the surface-level issue, such as the dishwasher or a lost scarf, but rather deeper underlying concerns such as power dynamics, unmet needs, lack of respect and poor communication. Sometimes, we repeat arguments as adults that we witnessed between our parents. Sometimes, we have fights with our partners that we would have liked to have had with our parents, but couldn't because we were too afraid.

In this case, you can see that for one partner the lost scarf raised feelings of not being cared for or thought about as a child, being overlooked, ignored, forgotten. The lost scarf represented the actions of a careless parent who didn't attend to their child. When our needs aren't met as children, we can often expect our partners to fill in the gaps. Next time you are upset with your partner, think about your upset and where it comes from. *Is it really about the dishwasher?*

Repetition Compulsion

Why do we often end up with partners who seem to trigger hurts or wounds from the past? Freud believed that we all tend to seek out friends or partners in life who are familiar to us – usually people who are like our parents or siblings. Our early experiences shape our understanding of love, relationships and attachment.

Remember identification and internalization which we discussed in Chapter 3 (see page 55)? For good or bad we seek out this familiarity. This is fine if we had great parents and siblings. But what if we had a father who was unavailable or a mother who was critical? We may well seek out partners who are similarly unavailable or critical. What if we had a father like Scrooge had?

This is what Freud called the *repetition compulsion*. This is the unconscious tendency to repeatedly re-enact past negative experiences in order to understand and gain mastery over them. By choosing partners who trigger past wounds, we may be trying to create a different outcome from the original negative experience. For example, someone who had an emotionally distant father may go on to have adult relationships with partners who are repressed, distant or unavailable. Someone who had a mother who couldn't control her anger might find herself with partners who are manipulative or bullying. If as a child you had a parent who was serially unfaithful, you may tolerate a partner who cheats. In all of these cases, the individuals might not fully understand why they repeatedly choose partners who are distant, manipulative or unfaithful. Despite the disappointment of each relationship, they may continue to seek out similar dynamics.

We may also adopt traits, like 'people pleasing', for example, that we take into adulthood but which do not serve us well. In childhood, this may have helped us to cope with a dominating parent. But in adulthood it might well make us far too accepting, too 'nice' and therefore too easily taken advantage of. The problem with repetition compulsion is that it does not allow us to change because we just get caught up in the cycle. The only way out is to understand the original negative experience.

The answer to repetition compulsion is to gain awareness of our unconscious patterns. This can usually only be achieved with the help of a therapist. It is often very tricky to spot these patterns without the help of a professional. With help, we can then learn to treat ourselves with greater compassion, rather than repeating damaging and self-defeating behaviours.

'You've been criticizing yourself for years and it hasn't worked.
Try approving of yourself and see what happens.'

LOUISE L. HAY
Motivational speaker and author[47]

Self-compassion at Work

Work is such an important part of our lives. For many of us, it defines us. It can be a source of pride, a place where we learn, make friends and develop professionally.

When we make mistakes at work, we usually react in one of two ways: we become defensive and blame others, or we berate ourselves. Many of us are professional perfectionists who believe we have to get things right the whole time. We are hard on ourselves, self-critical and judgemental of our performance. This can be good as it can spur us on to be better, to improve. But there is increasing evidence that being too self-critical can backfire and make us actually less effective at work. Beating yourself up isn't the answer.

Research shows that self-criticism, in excess, is counter-productive.[48] It can demotivate us and stops us from achieving our goals. Remember the 'fight or flight' response described in Chapter 2? When we are constantly self-critical, we put our bodies and minds into a constant high-stress-alert state.

Research has also shown that self-criticism rewires our brain's neurocircuitry, making negative self-talk more habitual. This can lead to loss of self-esteem, negative perfectionism and procrastination.

American psychology professor Serena Chen has studied self-compassion in relation to professional growth. She believes that people who are kinder to themselves are more likely to have a growth mindset. By this she means that they are able to view their professional skills as malleable, not fixed. This allows them to react more positively when they suffer a setback at work because they have the capacity to believe that they can improve. As a result, even in the face of negative feedback, they believe that with hard work they can make positive changes.[49]

Writing in the *Harvard Business Review*, Professor Chen states that having a realistic view of our strengths and limitations is crucial for self-improvement. 'When people treat themselves with compassion', she writes, 'they are better able to arrive at realistic self-appraisals, which is the foundation for improvement. They are also more motivated to work on their weaknesses rather than think "What's the point?" and to summon the grit required to enhance skills and change bad habits.'[50]

Professor Chen also believes that self-compassion, over time, allows people to choose more authentic roles for themselves at work, rather than striving for perfection in jobs that they hate or remaining in workplaces they find dull or unsatisfying. This is because they think they are worth it!

HOW TO BE MORE SELF-COMPASSIONATE AT WORK

- Build up a tolerance to small mistakes by learning a new hobby or skill, where you will make mistakes simply because you are a beginner.
- Challenge your critical inner voice. Notice when you are self-critical and change the voice to one of a kind friend.
- Acknowledge your limits.
- Recognize you can't be perfect. Let go of perfectionism.
- Ask for help when you need it.
- Set achievable goals, not unrealistic ones.
- Be kind to yourself after difficult conversations.
- Learn from your mistakes. Instead of beating yourself up, use your mistakes as opportunities to learn.
- Celebrate your professional achievements, however small.
- Keep a gratitude journal.

CASE STUDY: CHRIS

Chris was a maths teacher at a secondary school who was struggling to overcome the end of his marriage. He was dedicated to his students and passionate about fostering a love of maths in them. Like all teachers, he often found himself juggling numerous responsibilities, including marking, preparing lessons and attending parents' evenings.

The summer term was always particularly busy because of GCSE and A-Level exams and leavers' events. Chris was already struggling, as he had begun to open up in therapy about his marriage, something he had not really talked about at all with anyone. He found it helpful, but also overwhelming, as he felt he was only just starting to grieve the loss of a long relationship. At school he just pushed through, thinking if he just worked harder he would be fine.

One week, the headteacher asked Chris to help with interviews for a new head of physics. Chris was already swamped with marking, two parents' evenings, a reception for new parents and other academic commitments. But he felt he should say yes. Soon, however, he realized he couldn't do it all and he fell into a frenzy of negative self-talk.

After taking some time to reflect, Chris was able to remind himself that he was a dedicated teacher and it was actually okay to say no to some things, that working himself to exhaustion didn't help anyone, least of all himself. He wondered if his personal distress over his marriage might be something he could share with his headteacher. Chris did speak to his headteacher, and admitted he was overwhelmed by grief and felt he couldn't do the physics interviews. Fortunately, Chris's headteacher was understanding and compassionate and found someone else to help conduct the interviews.

Being compassionate towards yourself at work isn't about overlooking or disregarding your mistakes, or being lazy or complacent. Instead, it's about accepting when you've made a mistake and choosing to learn from it or, as in Chris's case, acknowledging your limitations.

EXERCISE: BOX BREATHING

This simple breathing technique has been shown to quiet an anxious mind, lower blood pressure, improve sleep and support overall mental well-being. It is a useful tool when you are having a stressful time at work or with your partner, as it can be done quickly wherever you are. Picture a box and follow these steps:

1. Inhale through the nose for four seconds. Picture yourself travelling up one side of the box.
2. Hold your breath for four seconds and visualize travelling along the top of the box.
3. Exhale for four seconds at the same rate that you inhaled as you visualize travelling down the side of the box.
4. Hold the lungs in an empty state for four seconds as you visualize travelling along the bottom of the box.

Repeat this sequence four times, which will bring you to around one minute of controlled breathing. Work your way up to five- or ten-minute sessions as you become more comfortable.

A Word on Shame

We all feel shame at times. It is a painful emotion that stems from believing that others see us in a negative light. It is a feeling of humiliation or embarrassment caused by believing we have done something immoral or dishonorable, such as telling a lie. It can also be a feeling that something is wrong with us, that we are essentially unloveable.

'Healing shame is about learning to see yourself with compassion and learning to love yourself, no matter what.'

TERRY REAL

Licensed Independent Clinical Social Worker (LICSW), Author of *Us: Getting Past You & Me to Build a More Loving Relationship*[51]

Shame is a self-critical emotion. It involves negatively judging ourselves when we believe we have failed to live up to certain standards. Shame provokes feelings of intense discomfort, and often a desire to hide from everything and everyone.

WAYS TO COMBAT SHAME

Acknowledge and name it. Naming shame can help you to be more aware of it so that it does not dominate you or pull you into a negative spiral.

- Remind yourself that shame is a universal emotion that everyone experiences at some point.
- Try to respond to your feelings of shame with self-compassion. Forgive yourself.
- Share your feelings of shame with a partner or friend.
- Remember that you are not defined by your shame and that the mistake or flaw which led to you feeling ashamed is not a reflection of who you are.
- Learn from your shame. Use it as a helpful lesson.

Shame often arises from a sense of scrutiny or ridicule from people who are more powerful than us. For example, children will feel ashamed if their parents express contempt for them.

Some shame is healthy and even necessary. For example it would be right to feel ashamed if you insulted someone for no reason, or humiliated a child or engaged in a criminal activity. This type of shame helps us to see when we have done something wrong. In evolutionary terms, shame allowed our ancestors to adhere to cultural rules and norms.

But shame, if persistent, can often be internalized so that we begin to see ourselves as terribly flawed. This can lead to low self-esteem. In some cases, shame can become chronic, contributing to mental-health challenges like depression or anxiety.

Self-compassion is crucial in counteracting shame. When we practise self-compassion, we allow ourselves to be less than perfect and we try not to judge ourselves too harshly. This can help to reduce the internalization of shame.

Key Takeaways

- Self-compassion is important in our romantic relationships and always makes us happier within a couple. It generally means we are more forgiving, more trusting, kinder and better at resolving arguments.
- Arguments in romantic relationships are never usually about surface issues, like who last emptied the dishwasher. They are usually related to deeper, unresolved issues such as poor communication, unmet needs or unequal power dynamics.
- Freud believed we can unconsciously seek out partners who trigger past wounds. He called this repetition compulsion – the unconscious tendency to repeatedly re-enact past negative experiences in order to gain mastery over them.
- Research shows that negative self-talk and criticism at work actually hinders progress. Self-compassion allows us to react more positively when we suffer a professional setback, giving us the belief that we can improve.
- Shame is a strong self-critical emotion which can be lessened with self-compassion.

CHAPTER SEVEN

How Can We Be More Compassionate to Others?

Here's a reminder of why compassion is important. The giving and receiving of compassion has major beneficial impacts on our physical and mental well-being. It makes us and the people around us happier and healthier. To be a compassionate person means to be mindful of what is going on around you, how it affects yourself and others, and what you can do to make things better. In this chapter we will look at barriers to compassion, such as compassion collapse and psychological defences. It concludes with some easy tips on how you can be more compassionate.

Barriers to Compassion

Let's look at what can prevent us from being compassionate to others. We learnt in Chapter 1 the components of compassion: non-judgement, being able to manage our own distress, sensitivity, sympathy and empathy. If we lack or struggle with any of these, it will be hard for us to be compassionate. We may also struggle if we grow up without any role models for compassion. Let's look at some other important barriers:

Anger & Resentment

Anger blocks our ability to empathize with others. When we are angry, it becomes difficult to understand other people's perspectives or the reasons behind their actions. Resentment stops us from forgiving. The psychoanalyst Ron Britton has highlighted how forgiveness requires a psychological shift, where an individual moves beyond their own anger and learns to understand the motives and suffering of the other person involved.[52] Forgiveness is not just an act of releasing the anger but also a recognition of the person who hurt you as a flawed human being with their own struggles.

Lack of Generosity

Remember Scrooge? He was the epitome of meanness. When we lack generosity, we are primarily focused on ourselves and much less likely to see or care about the suffering or needs of those around us. This, of course, makes compassion almost impossible. We perhaps all need to take a look at our inner Scrooge from time to time.

Lack of Self-compassion

When we are hard and critical towards ourselves, it becomes much more complicated for us to extend feelings of care and compassion to others.

Defences Such as Projection, Splitting, Denial & Repression

Psychological defences are unconscious strategies that help people manage anxiety, conflict or emotional pain. They are essentially protective, in that they help us avoid things we don't want to think about or deal with. But they often interfere with our ability to show compassion.

Projection is a psychoanalytic concept which describes how someone displaces their feelings, thoughts or traits onto someone else. This happens typically when someone has unacceptable or uncomfortable feelings they cannot tolerate. They can then distance themselves from the distressing emotions that they don't want to address. Essentially, what is internal is then seen as external.

For example, someone who may have a lot of repressed anger might spend a lot of time accusing others of being angry. Or someone who feels worthless might habitually criticize other people. The concept of projection emerged from Freud's work on defence mechanisms and was further refined by his daughter, Anna Freud.

When we project our thoughts, fears, anxieties or anger onto someone else, we no longer see them for who they are. It distorts our perception of them and prevents us from understanding them. It goes without saying that feeling compassion for that person then becomes problematic.

The concept of splitting was developed by British psychoanalyst Melanie Klein, who believed it developed in infancy as a way to protect the baby from anxiety, conflict and overwhelming emotions. Klein stated very young children view people in extreme terms, either as completely good or completely bad. This is because they are unable to hold contradictory feelings. As we mature we learn to integrate this black and white thinking and to understand that we, as well as those around us, can be both good and bad at the same time (see page 52 for more on this).

If splitting persists into adulthood, though, it can cause problems in regulating emotions and relationships. For example, if your best friend of many years no longer wants to see you because you upset him or her in a minor way, this may be because the friend saw you as perfect and cannot tolerate any perceived 'badness' in you. Your friend shifts from seeing you as all good to all bad, ignoring all the good aspects of your friendship. This binary view stems from a lack of compassion.

Compassion Collapse

Compassion collapse or fatigue refers to a phenomenon where people experience a diminished ability to feel compassion when confronted with large-scale or overwhelming suffering.

Charles Figley, an American psychologist and chair in Disaster Mental Health at Tulane University, defines compassion fatigue as 'a state of exhaustion and dysfunction, biologically, physiologically and emotionally, as a result of prolonged exposure to compassion stress.'[53] Symptoms include exhaustion, depression, anxiety, numbness and lack of empathy. Compassion fatigue mostly affects people working in challenging professions such as healthcare and the military. But it can also affect the general population, especially when we are subjected to constant news cycles which feature wars, climate change and extremist views.

The term 'compassion collapse' was first coined in 1992 by Carla Joinson to describe the negative impact on hospital nurses from their repeated exposure to sick patients.[54] However, Samuel Moyn, Professor of Law and History at Yale University, believes compassion fatigue goes back a long way. 'Compassion fatigue is as old as compassion,' he has written.[55] Here are some tips on how to combat compassion collapse:

- Focus on small things you can do, rather than allowing yourself to feel overwhelmed by the bigger picture. If you feel overwhelmed about climate change, think about doing small things such as planting a tree.
- Practise self-compassion so that you focus on staying emotionally balanced. Stop watching 24-hour news and try to refrain from 'doom scrolling'.
- Find groups or communities you could join that engage in compassionate action.
- Practise gratitude: focus on things that are good in the world.

How to Be Compassionate to Others

Everything you have learned so far in this book will help you be compassionate to others. Let's recap, and then look at some tips, rules and exercises that can help you become a more compassionate partner, parent and colleague.

The Components of Compassion

We know that to show compassion we need to be non-judgemental, sympathetic, empathetic, sensitive, willing to act and able to tolerate our own difficult feelings. All of these components will give us a greater ability to respond to someone else who is suffering, even if it is someone we don't like or someone who drives us to distraction.

The Physiology of Compassion

We know we can calm ourselves down in times of stress by practising self-compassion. When we learn to manage and control our challenging emotions, we are much better able to offer compassion to others.

The Development of Compassion

We know that the environment in which we grew up can affect our ability to be compassionate to others. Examining our childhoods, our parents, how our superego and attachment style may have developed and what we internalized from our caregivers will help us become more aware of the way we behave. Becoming more aware of how we behave allows us to be more in control of how we respond to others. It gives us a choice to respond in a compassionate way.

Thinking & Behaving Compassionately

We can try to train ourselves to think, reason and behave compassionately if we become more aware of what we are thinking. If we are in control of our thoughts, then we can choose to direct them towards being compassionate.

Learning Self-compassion

If we can learn to be self-compassionate, we are much more likely to show compassion to others. A crucial component of self-compassion is learning common humanity – that everyone fails.

EXERCISE: LOVING-KINDNESS MEDITATION

Buddhists have been directing compassion outwards for thousands of years by practising loving-kindness, or *metta*, meditations. The goal of *metta* meditation is to cultivate kindness for all beings. In a typical loving-kindness practice, we might focus on generating feelings of compassion for ourselves and then gradually expand our circle of compassion outwards to encompass loved ones, difficult people and finally all sentient beings. Here is a loving kindness meditation you can try:

1. Slowly focus on these words and repeat them silently three times: 'May I be happy, may I be healthy, may I be safe, may I live with ease.' (You can also swap out these words for whichever ones you'd like, for example: 'May I be peaceful, may I be free from suffering.')
2. Now picture a loved one and send feelings of loving-kindness to them as you repeat the same words three times: 'May you be happy, may you be healthy, may you be safe, may you live with ease.'
3. Focus on a person you are finding difficult at the moment or don't like, whether this is someone in your family, a work colleague or a stranger. Keep them in mind as you repeat these words three times: 'May they be happy, may they be healthy, may they be safe, may they live with ease.'
4. Finally, imagine loving-kindness spreading outwards to encompass all living things on the planet. Then repeat three times: 'May all be happy, may all be healthy, may all be safe, may all live with ease.'

How Can I Be a More Compassionate Partner?

In relationships, compassion means being aware of our partner's feelings, needs and struggles. It also means making an effort to engage with whatever is bothering them. We know from studies that when we behave in a compassionate way towards our partners we strengthen our relationship. Research shows that couples who cultivate compassion for one another report greater satisfaction in their relationships and are more likely to stay together.[56] It isn't always easy, but here are some tips:

- Be supportive when your partner is struggling. Make an effort to understand their problems and find out how you can help.
- Try to forgive mistakes. Our partners don't usually do things deliberately to hurt us. Usually they hurt us innocently, through lapses in judgement or tiredness or because they are stressed. Remember who your partner is.
- Don't idealize them or expect them to be someone they are not. Speak to each other in a compassionate way.
- Don't shout or swear or threaten violence or divorce when you are angry.
- Try to understand your partner's perspective, even if you don't agree with it.
- Practise patience.
- Have a weekly check-in with each other.
- Agree to stop arguing after fifteen minutes.

GENERAL RULES FOR SHOWING COMPASSION TO OTHERS

- Listen to what people are saying to you and try to understand the feelings behind their words. Are they putting on a brave face when actually they are really sad, for example?
- Be sensitive to people's words and actions. Notice what is going on.
- Practise empathy. Put yourself in other people's shoes: try to understand their situation and emotions, imagining how you would feel if you were in their position.
- Don't judge. Be encouraging.
- Show kindness through your actions.
- Practise self-awareness.
- Be forgiving.
- Express gratitude.
- Accept people for who they are.

How Can I Be a More Compassionate Parent?

We know how important parents are in shaping and developing their children's compassion. No one wants to be like Scrooge's father. Yet parenting is one of the toughest jobs we will ever have. It requires endless patience, tolerance, understanding and empathy. It is always a challenge. One of the most important things we can do as parents is to acknowledge our limitations – that we won't always get it right and be kind to ourselves when we make mistakes. This is not a how-to-parent book, but here are some general rules for compassionate parenting:

- Provide unconditional love, warmth and affection.
- Listen to what your children say to you, sympathize and empathize with their feelings, whether positive or negative.
- Teach your children how to be compassionate by modelling compassionate behaviour.
- Never label children.
- Remember that change can stimulate strong emotions in children.
- Communicate openly and honestly.
- Discipline in a positive way.
- Never use violence.
- Teach respect.
- Teach your children to take responsibility for their actions.
- Practise self-compassion.
- Encourage acts of kindness.

How Can I Be More Compassionate at Work?

The places where we work have an emotional component to them. We make friends at work, we show off our skills at work, we sometimes fail at work. When colleagues treat each other with compassion it contributes to a positive and supportive professional environment. This in turn improves our sense of satisfaction at work, as well as engendering a sense of loyalty to our workplace. A positive work environment can reduce our anxiety and make us more resilient to work stress. Here are some tips:

- Help colleagues who are struggling either professionally or personally.
- Acknowledge your colleagues' achievements.
- Communicate honestly.
- Offer support without judgement.
- Acknowledge your colleagues' perspectives.
- Be inclusive. Don't leave people out.
- Respect and encourage your colleagues' work-life balance.
- Practise patience.
- Be understanding during stressful times.

How Can I Be More Compassionate to People I Don't Like?

Often, we find it hardest to be compassionate towards those who challenge us the most, whether these people are members of our extended family, colleagues or even strangers. It is possible, though, and even desirable because it helps us maintain our *own* well-being too. Here are some tips:

- Let go of judgement.
- Don't take their words or actions personally. Often bad behaviour from others is a reflection of their own internal struggles and has nothing to do with you.
- Understand your feelings towards the person and know that it is permissible to feel annoyed or upset with them, while not allowing these feelings to dominate you.
- Try to understand their perspective.
- Set boundaries. Don't sacrifice your own well-being for a tricky friend or family member. You don't *have* to have your selfish aunt to stay for a week.
- Don't hold on to anger, resentment or grudges. Consider whether the person you dislike is actually triggering something significant in you, such as jealousy or fear.

Final Word

Compassion is hard. It may not work immediately and you may find yourself going backwards every so often. It is an ongoing practice, a lifelong way of behaving, one that we can choose to embrace every day with every interaction, no matter how big or small.

It isn't a magic recipe. Some people or situations will challenge you and make you lose all sense of compassion. You may not always have all the answers or know exactly how to act in every situation. But you do have the power to choose how you respond to your own feelings and to the people around you.

If you want to take things further, you should consider working with a therapist who will help you learn to be compassionate to yourself. But everything you have read in this book you can think about or practise at home.

Remember, the more we practise compassion, the more it becomes a natural part of who we are. The more compassion we cultivate in our lives, the more it can transform the world around us, too.

Key Takeaways

- There are many barriers to compassion, such as anger, lack of generosity and self-compassion, and psychological defences such as projection, splitting, denial and repression.
- Projection is a psychological defence in which we displace our own intolerable feelings onto someone else.
- Splitting occurs when someone perceives themselves or others as either all good or all bad, with no nuance or middle ground.
- Compassion collapse is when someone is unable to feel compassion in the face of overwhelming suffering.
- The more we practise compassion, the more it becomes a natural part of who we are.

Endnotes

1.   The Dalai Llama. (1999). *The Art of Happiness: A Handbook for Living*. London: Hodder & Stoughton.

2.   Dickens, C. (1843). *A Christmas Carol*. London: Chapman & Hall.

3.   Vance, J.D. (January 2025). Fox News.

4.   Pope Francis. (February 2025). 'Letter of the Holy Father to the bishops of the United States of America'. https://press.vatican.va/content/salastampa/en/bollettino/pubblico/2025/02/11/250211e.html.

5.   Ibid 1.

6.   The Dalai Lama. 'Compassion and the Individual'. www.dalailama.com/messages/compassion-and-human-values/compassion.

7.   Gilbert, P. (2010). *The Compassionate Mind*. London: Constable.

8.   Weng, H.Y., Fox, A.S., Shackman, A.J., Stodola, D.E., Caldwell J.Z.K., Olson, M.C., Rogers, G.M. and Davidson, R.J. (2013). 'Compassion training alters altruism and neural responses to suffering'. *Psychological Science*, Volume 24, Issue 7. doi: 10.1177/0956797612469537.

9.   Salzberg, S. (2017). *Real Love: The Art of Mindful Connection*. London: Pan Macmillan.

10. Mantelou, A. and Karakasidou, E. (2017). 'The Effectiveness of a Brief Self-Compassion Intervention Program on Self-Compassion, Positive and Negative Affect and Life Satisfaction'. *Psychology*. 8, 590-610. doi.org/10.4236/psych.2017.84038.

11. Gilbert, P. (2009). 'Introducing compassion-focused therapy'. *Advances in Psychiatric Treatment*. 15(3):199-208. doi:10.1192/apt.bp.107.005264.

12. Wang, S. (2005) in Mongrain, M., Chin, J. M. and Shapira, L. M. (2010). 'Practicing compassion increases happiness and self-esteem'. *Journal of Happiness Studies*, 12 (6), 963-981.

13. Dunn, E.W., Aknin, L.B. and Norton, M.I. (2008). 'Spending money on others promotes happiness'. *Science*. Mar 21;319(5870):1687-8. doi:10.1126/science.1150952. Erratum in: *Science*. 2009 May 29;324(5931):1143. PMID: 18356530.

14. Aknin, L.B., Hamlin J.K. and Dunn. E.W. (2012). 'Giving Leads to Happiness in Young Children'. *PLoS One*. 7(6):e39211. doi:10.1371/journal.pone.0039211.

15. Konrath, S., Fuhrel-Forbis, A., Lou, A., and Brown, S. (2012). 'Motives for volunteering are associated with mortality risk in older adults'. *Health Psychology*, *31*(1), 87–96. doi.org/10.1037/a0025226.

16. Moll, J., Krueger, F., Zahn, R., Pardini, M., de Oliveira-Souza, R. and Grafman, J. (2006). 'Human fronto-mesolimbic networks guide decisions about charitable donation'. *Proc Natl Acad Sci*. 17;103(42):15623-8. doi:10.1073/pnas.0604475103.

17. Cacioppo, J.T., Cacioppo, S., Capitanio, J.P. and Cole, S.W. (2015). 'The neuroendocrinology of social isolation'. *Annual Review of Psychology*. Vol. 66:733-767. doi.org/10.1146/annurev-psych-010814-015240.

18. Ibid 15.

19. Brown, S., Nesse, R., Vinokur, A. and Smith, D. (2003). 'Providing social support may be more beneficial than receiving it: results from a prospective study of mortality'. *Psychol Sci*. Jul;14(4):320-7. doi:10.1111/1467-9280.14461.

20. Seppala, E. (2014). 'Connectedness & Health: The Science of Social Connection'. The Center for Compassion and Altruism Research and Education. ccare.stanford.edu/uncategorized/connectedness-health-the-science-of-social-connection-infographic/

21. Fowler, J. and Christakis, N. (2008). 'Dynamic spread of happiness in a large social network: longitudinal analysis over 20 years in the Framingham Heart Study'. *BMJ* 2008;337:a2338.

22. Brown, B. (2018). *Dare to Lead*. London: Penguin.

23. Neff, K. (2011). *Self-Compassion: The Proven Power of Being Kind to Yourself*. New York: HarperCollins.

24. Han, A. and Kim, T.H. (2023). 'Effects of Self-Compassion Interventions on Reducing Depressive Symptoms, Anxiety, and Stress: A Meta-Analysis'. *Mindfulness* (N Y). Jun 5:1–29. Online ahead of print. doi: 10.1007/s12671-023-02148-x; Raque, T.L., Lamphere, B., Motzny, C., Kauffmann, J., Ziemer, K., and Haywood, S. (2023). 'Pathways by Which Self-Compassion Improves Positive Body Image: A Qualitative Analysis'. *Behavioural Sciences* Nov 16;13(11):939. doi: 10.3390/bs13110939.

25. The Center for Compassion and Altruism Research and Education, Stanford University. 'Mission & Vision'. www.ccare.stanford.edu/about/mission-vision/.

26. Darwin, C. (1871). *The Descent of Man, and Selection in Relation to Sex*. London: John Murray.

27. Dickel, D.N. and Doran, G.H. (1989). 'Severe neural tube defect syndrome from the early archaic of Florida'. doi.org/10.1002/ajpa.1330800306.

28. Spikins, P. A., Rutherford, H. E., and Needham, A. P. (2010). 'From Homininity to Humanity: Compassion from the Earliest Archaics to Modern Humans'. *Time and Mind*, 3(3), 303–325. https://doi.org/10.2752/175169610X12754030955977.

29. McGonigal, K. (2016). *The Science of Compassion: A Modern Approach for Cultivating Empathy, Love and Connection*. Colorado: Sounds True Inc.

30. Ibid.

31. Hoffman, M.L. (2001). 'Prosocial Behavior and Empathy: Developmental Processes' in Smelser, N.J. and Baltes, P.B. (ed.) *International Encyclopedia of the Social & Behavioral Sciences*, Pergamon, Pages 12230-12233, doi.org/10.1016/B0-08-043076-7/01739-3.

32. Klein, M., Heimann, P., Isaacs, S. and Riviere, J. (1952). *Developments in Psychoanalysis*. London: Routledge.

33. Piaget, J. and Inhedler, B. (1969). *The Psychology of the Child*. New York: Basic Books; Piaget, J. (1968). *Six Psychological Studies*. Translated by Tenzer, A. and Elkind, D. New York: Vintage Books.

34. Winnicott, D. (2005). *Playing and Reality*. London: Routledge.

35. Bowlby, J. (1978). 'Attachment theory and its therapeutic implications'. *Adolescent Psychiatry*. 6, 5–33.

36. Aurelius, M. (161–180 CE). *Meditations*.

37. Shakespeare, W. (1599–1601). *Hamlet*. Act 2, Scene 2.

38. Raes, F., Pommier, E., Neff, K.D. and Van Gucht, D. (2011). 'Construction and Factorial Validation of a Short Form of the Self-Compassion Scale'. *Clinical Psychology & Psychotherapy*. 18, 250-255. doi: 10.1002/cpp.702.

39. Neff, K. self-compassion.org.

40. Neff, K. self-compassion.org/exercises/exercise-2-self-compassion-break/.

41. Attributed to Mark Twain. (1934). *Reader's Digest*.

42. Breines, J.G. and Chen, S. (2012). 'Self-compassion increases self-improvement motivation'. Pers Soc Psychol Bull. Sep;38(9):1133-43.

43. Neff, K. and Germer, G. (2018). *The Mindful Self-Compassion Workbook*. New York: The Guildford Press.

44. Martin-Luther-Universität Halle-Wittenberg. (2024). 'Couples: Caring for oneself can lead to happier relationships – on both sides'. *Science Daily*. www.sciencedaily.com/releases/2024/01/240123122142.htm.

45. Real, T. (2022). *Us: Getting Past You & Me to Build a More Loving Relationship*. Pennsylvania: Rodale Books.

46. Neff, K.D. and Beretvas S.N. (2012). 'The Role of Self-compassion in Romantic Relationships'. *Self and Identity*, doi:10.1080/15298868.2011.639548.

47. Hay, Louise L. (1984). *You Can Heal Your Life*. California: Hay House.

48. Powers, T. A., Koestner, R., and Zuroff, D. C. (2007). 'Self-criticism, goal motivation, and goal progress.' *Journal of Social and Clinical Psychology*, 26(7), 826–840. doi.org/10.1521/jscp.2007.26.7.826

49. Breines, J. & Chen, S. (2012). 'Self-Compassion Increases Self-Improvement Motivation'. Personality and Social Psychology Bulletin 38(9): 1133-43. doi:10.1177/0146167212445599.

50. Chen, S. (September 2018). 'Give Yourself a Break: The Power of Self-Compassion'. *Harvard Business Review*.

51. Real, T. (January 2025). www.instagram.com/p/DFGQdbSMfKo/1048735693724237/.

52. Britton, R. and Novakovic, A. (Ed). (2023). *Psychoanalytic Approaches to Forgiveness and Mental Health*. London: Routledge.

53. Figley, C. R. (Ed.). (1995). *Compassion Fatigue: Coping with Secondary Traumatic Stress Disorder in Those Who Treat the Traumatized*. New York: Routledge.

54. Joinson, C. (1992). 'Coping with compassion fatigue.' *Nursing.* 22(4):116-120.

55. Moyn, S. Quoted in (2018), 'Is compassion fatigue ineviatable in an age of 24-hour news?'. *The Guardian*. https://www.theguardian.com/news/2018/aug/02/is-compassion-fatigue-inevitable-in-an-age-of-24-hour-news.

56. Fehr, B., Harasymchuk, C., and Sprecher, S. (2014). 'Compassionate love in romantic relationships: A review and some new findings'. *Journal of Social and Personal Relationships*, 31(5), 575–600. doi.org/10.1177/0265407514533768.

Further Reading

Gilbert, P. (2010). *The Compassionate Mind*. London: Constable.

Gilbert, P. (ed.) (2017). *Compassion Concepts, Research and Applications*. London: Routledge.

Irons, C. and Beaumont, A. (2017). *The Compassionate Mind Workbook*. London: Robinson.

McGonigal, K. (2016). *The Science of Compassion: A Modern Approach for Cultivating Empathy, Love and Connection*. Colorado: Sounds True.

Neff, K. (2011). *Self-Compassion: The Proven Power of Being Kind to Yourself*. New York: HarperCollins.

Neff, K. and Germer, G. (2018). *The Mindful Self-Compassion Workbook*. New York: The Guildford Press.

Schweikert, C. (2023). *The Compassion Remedy*. Rhode Island: WorldChangers Media.

Acknowledgements

This book would not have been written without the help, encouragement and support of the following people.

Sophie Lazar, Commissioning Editor at Quarto, for asking and then trusting me to write it. And Katerina Menhennet, who was a kind and patient editor.

My kind and generous friends who read early chapter drafts, suggested improvements and made me think a little deeper: Anna Blundy, Sophie Arie, Sarah Philps, Johnna Wellesley, Sally Peck, Alan Philps, Louise Hayman, Kate Mills and Flo Bayley.

My compassionate supervisor, Dr Sharon Numa, who elevated the chapters and made them wiser.

My family: Thais Warren who appraised early drafts and was, with Callum Printsmith, a great cheerleader. Greg Warren and Sanna Aizad who helped me with research papers and read the science.

Most thanks are due to my husband, Marcus Warren, who edited, cajoled, informed and encouraged me throughout, and to my son, Edward Warren, who put up with it all.

About the Author

Sally Warren is a former journalist who covered major home and foreign news stories for *The Daily Telegraph* for more than a decade. She re-trained as an adult psychoanalytic psychotherapist after leaving newspapers to start a family. She has a private practice in central London and is a therapist for The Mind Field, a global online therapy platform for journalists and humanitarians. She continues to write on psychoanalytic subjects for various publications and was recently appointed a trustee of the British Psychotherapy Foundation, where she trained. She is married with a son and two stepchildren and lives in central London.

Index

The *Find Your Path* Series

Find Your Path books shed light on a range of common mental-health struggles, from depression to imposter syndrome, and offer powerful techniques for navigating life's inevitable ups and downs.

Find Your Path through Anxiety: Mindful techniques to help you find ease (2025)

Find Your Path through Depression: Mindful techniques for dark times (2025)

Find Your Path through Imposter Syndrome: Powerful techniques to help you see your worth (2025)

Find Your Path to Resilience: Powerful techniques to build emotional strength (2025)